14.95

Killey's Fractures of the l

D0130456

Killey's Fractures of the Mandible

Fourth Edition

Peter Banks MB BS (Lond) FDS RCS (Eng)
Consultant in Oral and Maxillofacial Surgery, Plastic and
Maxillofacial Unit, Queen Victoria Hospital, East Grinstead,
West Sussex; Royal East Sussex Hospital, Hastings, East Sussex;
Kent County Ophthalmic and Aural Hospital, Maidstone, Kent

Civil Consultant in Oral and Maxillofacial Surgery to the Royal
Air Force

Honorary Senior Lecturer and Consultant, Department of Oral
Surgery, Institute of Dental Surgery, Eastman Dental Hospital,
London

Formerly Consultant Oral Surgeon, Addenbrooke's Hospital,
Cambridge, and Peterborough District Hospital

Wright

Wright
is an imprint of Butterworth–Heinemann Ltd

 PART OF REED INTERNATIONAL P.L.C.

OXFORD LONDON GUILDFORD BOSTON MUNICH NEWDELHI
SINGAPORE SYDNEY TOKYO TORONTO WELLINGTON

All rights reserved. No part of this publication may be reproduced in any material
form (including photocopying or storing it in any medium by electronic means and
whether or not transiently or incidentally to some other use of this publication)
without the written permission of the copyright owner except in accordance with
the provisions of the Copyright, Designs and Patents Act 1988 or under the terms
of a licence issued by the Copyright Licensing Agency Ltd, 33–34 Alfred Place,
London, England WC1E 7DP. Applications for the copyright owner's written
permission to reproduce any part of this publication should be addressed to the
Publishers.

Warning: The doing of an unauthorised act in relation to a copyright work may
result in both a civil claim for damages and criminal prosecution.

This book is sold subject to the Standard Conditions of Sale of Net Books and may
not be re-sold in the UK below the net price given by the Publishers in their current
price list.

© **Butterworth–Heinemann Ltd, 1991**

First edition, 1967
Second edition, 1971
Revised reprint, 1974
Reprinted, 1977
Reprinted, 1980
Third edition, 1983
Reprinted, 1985
Reprinted, 1988
Fourth edition, 1991

British Library Cataloguing in Publication Data

Killey, H. C.
  Killey's fractures of the mandible.–4th ed.
  —(A Dental Practitioners Handbook)
  1. Jaws–fractures
  I. Title
  II. Banks, Peter   II. Series
  617′.15′6   RD526

ISBN 0-7236-0708-7

Composition by Genesis Typesetting, Laser Quay, Rochester, Kent
Printed in Great Britain by BPCC Wheatons Ltd, Exeter

Preface to the fourth edition

The text for the fourth edition of this handbook has been extensively revised to reflect current practice. In so doing every attempt has been made to preserve the original author's intention – to provide an outline of the principles of treatment of fractures of the mandible for students and interested general practitioners.

Examination of the literature of the past 10 years reveals a substantial change in the pattern of facial injuries. In most countries of the world there has been a decline in road traffic trauma and an increase in urban violence. Traditional methods of treatment by the routine application of intermaxillary fixation have come into question. Improvements in the technical specification of miniaturized bone plates have led to much more widespread use of direct osteosynthesis obviating uncomfortable and often debilitating periods of intermaxillary fixation.

Modern methods of treatment demand greater surgical skills and established simpler techniques still have their place. An attempt has been made to place all these methods of treatment in their proper perspective. There remain certain types of injury, notably fractures of the condylar region, where the results of treatment fall short of the ideal. Where current knowledge is incomplete the relevant current literature has been emphasized.

Every effort has been made to keep this edition as short as its predecessors and this inevitably means some sacrifice of desirable illustrations. A number of additional diagrams and photographs have, however, been included and a few eliminated. It is hoped the new edition will continue to be a useful guide to examination candidates and those taking their first steps towards specialization.

P.B.

Acknowledgements

I am particularly grateful to Mr A. E. Brown, FDS FRCS for many of the line drawings which appear as Figures 2.1, 2.8, 3.6, 6.4, 6.5, 6.13, 6.15, 6.16, 6.17, 6.19, 6.30, 6.32, 6.34 and 8.2. I am also grateful to Mr Brown for allowing me to reproduce his method of fixation of a fractured condyle as illustrated in Figures 8.2 and 8.3. A number of other consultant colleagues have kindly allowed reproduction of photographs of cases under their care, particularly Mr M. D. Awty, Mr P. T. Blenkinsop and Dr J. Prein. Acknowledgements appear under the particular illustration. Dr Joachim Prein MD DDS, Professor of Maxillofacial Surgery, University Clinic of Basel, Switzerland has been most helpful in providing material to illustrate the AO plating system which is not widely used in the UK.

The additional photographs in this edition were all prepared by Mr Trevor Hill and Mr Andrew Hack in the Medical Illustrations Department, Queen Victoria Hospital, East Grinstead, and I would like to thank them both for their patient assistance. My final acknowledgement must be to the inventor of word processing.

Preface to the first edition

This outline of the diagnosis and treatment of fractures of the mandible is written as an introduction for students and as an aid to practitioners who treat mandibular fractures. It is not intended for the specialist maxillofacial surgeon, for in a book of this size it is impossible to cover the subject in the necessary detail. Technical data on splint construction have been omitted for the same reason and only the more important aspects of the techniques for immobilization of the fragments have been discussed. The complex subject of the so-called 'gunshot-type' fracture where there is loss of both hard and soft tissues has of necessity been dealt with very briefly.

At the Editor's request, references have been reduced to a minimum in an endeavour to make the text easier to read and the author apologizes for many important omissions. However, mention has been made in the Bibliography of the many excellent articles and books which have been consulted.

It is important that all dental surgeons should be familiar with the diagnosis and treatment of mandibular fractures. Such injuries are easy to diagnose and after a careful examination the clinician can correlate the physical signs with the underlying surgical anatomy, so visualizing the nature and extent of the bony injury. Radiology, if available, should never be omitted, but in most instances the radiographs should merely confirm the clinical findings.

The treatment of the majority of mandibular fractures should be well within the capabilities of any dental surgeon, for provided the fracture is accurately reduced and adequately immobilized for the requisite period of time, a satisfactory result can be confidently expected. It is important to avoid infection of the fracture line during healing and for this reason it is helpful to begin a prophylactic course of antibiotics as soon after injury as possible and to continue this treatment until shortly after reduction and immobilization of the fracture. This avoids infection of the fracture haematoma and experience has shown that it is much easier to prevent infection in this area than to treat an established infection. Reduction and immobilization should, of course, be effected as soon as the general medical condition of the patient permits.

H.C.K.

Contents

Chapter 1

Introduction

Fracture of the mandible occurs more frequently than any other fracture of the facial skeleton. It is the one serious facial bone injury that the average practising dental surgeon may expect to encounter, albeit on rare occasions, at his surgery. It is also a facial fracture which he may have the misfortune to cause as a complication of tooth extraction. The study of the management of mandibular fractures has therefore a real practical application which is not merely relevant to those studying for higher qualifications or pursuing a career in oral and maxillofacial surgery.

Fractures of the mandible may broadly be divided into two main groups:

1. Fractures with no gross comminution of the bone and without significant loss of hard or soft tissue.
2. Fractures with gross comminution of the bone and with extensive loss of both hard and soft tissue.

The majority of fractures fall into the first category. Those in the second group either result from missile injuries in war situations, industrial injuries involving machinery or major road accidents where there is direct injury from sharp objects moving at relatively high velocity. Although arbitrary, this broad division is useful because the general management of the second group is entirely different from the first both in the primary and in the reconstructive phases.

Aetiology

The causes of fracture of the mandible are chiefly road traffic accidents, interpersonal violence, falls, sporting injuries and industrial trauma. For 30 years after the Second World War road traffic accidents were found to be the major cause of fracture of the mandible accounting for between 35 and 60% of fractures of

1

the facial bones (Rowe and Killey, 1968; Vincent-Townend and Langdon, 1985). Perkins and Layton (1988) have recently reviewed the aetiology of maxillofacial injuries in general and have drawn attention to changes which have occurred during the last 10 years.

The relative importance of the various factors which affect the incidence of mandibular fractures is influenced by:

1. Geography.
2. Social trends.
3. Road traffic legislation.
4. Seasons.

Geography

Van Hoof *et al.* (1977) analysed the differing patterns of fracture of the facial skeleton in four European countries and observed considerable variation in the experience of the treatment centres from which they collected statistics. Injuries caused by fights were commoner in German urban areas than a unit in Holland, whereas the latter centre experienced a much higher incidence of road traffic trauma. In developing countries with a rapid increase in road traffic, motor vehicle trauma is the major cause of fractures (Adekeye, 1980).

Social trends

In urban areas in more recent years particularly, interpersonal violence has accounted for an increasing proportion of mandibular fractures (Ellis, Moos and El Attar, 1985; Eriksson and Willmar, 1987; Perkins and Layton, 1988). The relative incidence of other facial bone fractures and facial lacerations has been influenced by this trend, and in some urban centres zygomatic fractures are now more common than those of the mandible (Brook and Wood, 1983).

Road traffic legislation

Vehicle design has been influenced both by research and legislation and in some countries the use of seat belt restraint has been made compulsory in law. Seat belts have resulted in a dramatic decrease in injury in general and severe injury in particular (Thomas, 1990), and that trend has been reflected in the incidence of facial injury (Sabey, Grant and Hobbs, 1977).

Grattan and Hobbs (1985) have reported on the beneficial effects of improved car design and the use of seat belts. Enforced low speed limits do not appear to carry the same benefit as far as mandibular fractures are concerned (Olson *et al.*, 1982).

Seasons

Facial fractures show a seasonal variation in most temperate zones which reflects the increased traffic and increased urban violence during summer months and adverse road conditions in the presence of snow and ice in mid-winter.

Incidence

Mandibular fractures used to be more common than middle third injuries. In 1966 Schuchardt *et al.* found that the mandible was fractured either alone or in combination in no less than 2103 out of 2901 facial bone injuries. Oikarinen and Lindqvist (1975) studied 729 patients with multiple injuries sustained in traffic accidents; 11% of the patients had fractures of the facial bones. The most common facial fractures were in the mandible (61%), followed by the maxilla (46%), the zygoma (27%) and the nasal bones (19.5%).

The change in emphasis of the various aetiological factors outlined above is reflected in a reduction in the relative incidence of fractures of the mandible in more recent series. Brook and Wood (1983) have examined this trend over four decades in a retrospective study. During this period personal assaults increased by 75% and fractures of the zygoma became more common than fractures of the mandible, facts which may well be related. Although fracture of the mandibular condyle is the commonest site for mandibular fracture, the angle fracture is the most frequent site when only one fracture is present (Halazonetis, 1968; Ellis, Moos and El Attar, 1985). Among patients sustaining general injury as a result of personal assault, Shepherd *et al.* (1990) found that 83% of all fractures and 66% of all lacerations were facial.

Classification

There is no completely satisfactory classification of mandibular fractures. They may, however, be considered under three main headings:

1. Type of fracture
2. Site of fracture
3. Cause of fracture.

Type of fracture

Simple

These encompass closed linear fractures of the condyle, coronoid, ramus and edentulous body of the mandible. The greenstick fracture is a rare variant of the simple fracture and is found exclusively in children.

Compound

Fractures of the tooth-bearing portions of the mandible are nearly always compound into the mouth via the periodontal membrane and some severe injuries are compound through the overlying skin.

Comminuted

Direct violence to the mandible from penetrating sharp objects and missiles may cause limited or extensive comminution. Such fractures are usually compound and may be further complicated by bone and soft-tissue loss.

Pathological

Fractures are termed pathological when they result from minimal trauma to a mandible already weakened by a pathological condition such as osteomyelitis, neoplasms or generalized skeletal disease (Figure 1.1).

Site of fracture

The most useful classification for practical purposes is based on the anatomical location of the injury, for the signs and symptoms vary according to the site of fracture as does the treatment. Fractures of the mandible occur at the following sites (Figure 1.2):

(a) Dento-alveolar
(b) Condyle
(c) Coronoid
(d) Ramus

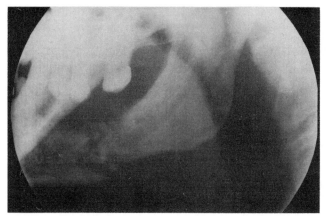

Figure 1.1 Pathological fracture of the mandible as a result of osteomyelitis following an extraction

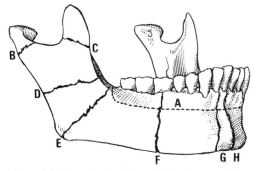

Figure 1.2 Classification of mandibular fracture sites. A, Dento-alveolar; B, Condylar; C, Coronoid; D, Ramus; E, Angle; F, Body; G, Parasymphysis; H, Symphysis

(e) Angle
(f) Body (molar and premolar areas)
(g) Parasymphysis
(h) Symphysis

The above represents a useful subdivision for consideration of linear fractures, but whenever there is even limited comminution such a classification becomes relatively meaningless.

Cause of fracture

The direction and type of impact is more important in considering fractures of the mandible than other areas of the facial skeleton as it is the factor which determines the pattern of mandibular injury. Fractures of the mandible result from:

(a) Direct violence
(b) Indirect violence
(c) Excessive muscular contraction.

Because of the shape of the mandible any direct violence to one area produces an indirect force of lesser dimension in another usually opposite part of the bone. This latter indirect violence may be sufficient to cause a second or third fracture as a result. From the point of view of treatment the pattern of the mandibular fracture is extremely important and can be considered under the following headings:

1. Unilateral fracture.
2. Bilateral fracture.
3. Multiple fracture.
4. Comminuted fracture.

Unilateral fracture

Unilateral fractures are usually single, but occasionally more than one fracture may be present on one side of the mandible and if this occurs there is often gross displacement of the fragments. A unilateral fracture of the body of the mandible is most frequently caused by direct violence but in the case of the weak condylar neck an indirect force may cause fracture while the site of direct impact remains intact.

Bilateral fracture

Bilateral fractures frequently occur from a combination of direct and indirect violence. Common bilateral fractures resulting from such a mechanism are those involving the angle and opposite condylar neck or the canine region and opposite angle. However, every possible combination and variation of the linear fractures already mentioned can occur bilaterally.

Multiple fracture

The same association of direct with indirect violence may give rise to multiple fractures. The most common multiple fracture is that caused by a fall on the mid-point of the chin resulting in fractures of the symphysis and both condyles. These fractures are commonly seen in epileptics, elderly patients who lose consciousness as a result of general disease, and occasionally in soldiers who faint on parade from which the fracture combination derives its name of 'guardsman' fracture.

Oikarinen and Malmstrom (1969), in a series of 600 mandibular fractures, found 49.1% were single, 39.9% had two fractures, 9.4% had three fractures, 1.2% had four fractures and 0.4% had more than four fractures.

Comminuted fractures

Comminution of a fracture site is almost invariably the result of considerable direct violence at the site of fracture as is commonly the case in war missile injuries (Figure 1.3). In civilian practice this

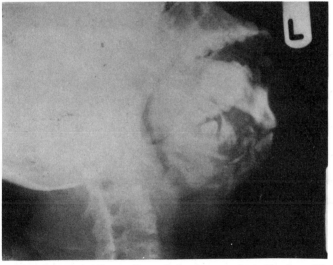

Figure 1.3 Lateral oblique radiograph showing comminuted fracture of the left body of the mandible following a medium velocity missile injury

degree of comminution is most common in the symphysis and parasymphyseal regions. Such fractures require special management and should therefore be considered in a category of their own. It is not unknown for severe missile injuries to cause comminution of the whole of the mandible from one condylar neck to the other.

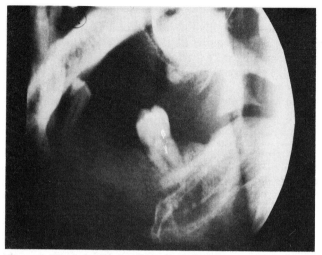

Figure 1.4 Lateral oblique radiograph showing fracture of the coronoid process with displacement due to pull of temporalis muscle

Fracture due to excessive muscular contracture

Occasionally fracture of the coronoid process occurs because of sudden reflex contracture of the temporalis muscle (Figure 1.4). Sudden muscular contracture may also be a factor in some fractures of the condylar neck.

Chapter 2

Surgical anatomy

The surgical anatomy of the mandible and adjacent structures is extremely important in understanding the pattern of fracture, the displacement of fractured bone ends and the factors necessary for uncomplicated healing. Although the mandible is embryologically a membrane bone its physical structure resembles a bent long bone with two articular cartilages and two nutrient arteries. This arch of cortico-cancellous bone projects down and forwards from the base of the skull and constitutes the strongest and most rigid component of the facial skeleton (Figure 2.1). It is, however, more commonly

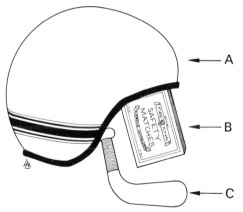

Figure 2.1 Diagrammatic representation of the strength of the bones of the skull and face. The 'match-box' structure of the midfacial skeleton cushions the effect of impact force B. Impact force A is transmitted directly to the brain producing the most severe injury. Impact force C is transmitted indirectly to the cranial base via the rigid structure of the mandible

fractured than the other bones of the face, a fact directly related to its prominent and exposed situation. Furthermore, unlike the 'matchbox-like' midfacial skeleton which readily absorbs direct trauma, blows to the mandible are transmitted directly to the base

9

of the skull through the temporomandibular articulation. This in turn means that relatively minor mandibular fractures may be associated with a surprising degree of head injury; hence the effectiveness of the boxer's knock-out punch.

Because of the associated head injury, fractures of the mandible may constitute a threat to the airway in the early period after injury. A patient whose level of consciousness is depressed is less able to protect his own airway from the embarrassment of blood, broken teeth and displaced dentures. Furthermore, bleeding into the floor of the mouth and base of the tongue causes swelling which may threaten to obstruct the oropharynx.

Mandibular fracture sites

The anatomical configuration of the mandible approximates to a rigid semi-circular link but with pinned joints at its free ends. Nahum (1975) measured the forces required to produce fractures of the facial bones in a series of cadaver experiments. Fracture of the maxilla occurred with forces as low as 140 lb whereas the lowest tolerance level of the mandible to frontal impact was 425 lb, which consistently produced fracture of the condylar neck. Fracture of the neck of the condyle can be regarded as a safety mechanism which protects the patient from the serious consequences of middle fossa fracture. Such a fracture can happen on rare occasions when the condylar head is driven through the glenoid fossa. Nahum observed that a frontal force of 800–900 lb was required to produce fracture of the symphysis and both condylar necks. He further demonstrated that the mandible was much more sensitive to lateral than to frontal impacts and concluded that a frontal impact at the symphysis was substantially cushioned by opening and retrusion of the jaw.

The teeth are most important in determining where fracture occurs. The long canine tooth and the part-erupted wisdom tooth both represent lines of relative weakness, and unerupted teeth such as premolars are important in the same way. Oikarinen and Malmstrom (1969) analysed 600 mandibular fractures by taking tracings from orthopantomographs. On analysis it was found that 33.4% of fractures took place in the subcondylar area, 17.4% at the angle, 6.7% were alveolar, 5.4% were in the ramus, 2.9% in the midline and 1.3% in the coronoid process, while 33.6% occurred in the body of the mandible mostly in the canine region.

Recent analysis of fracture patterns where urban interpersonal violence is the major cause show a reduced overall incidence in fractures of the condyle and an increase in the frequency of body fractures (Ellis, Moos and El Attar, 1985; Busuito, Smith and Robson, 1986). Similarly when the mandible is fractured at a single site only, the angle area seems most vulnerable (Halazonetis, 1968). The implication of these observations seems to be that the lesser direct violence from personal assaults tends to cause fracture at the usual point of impact on one side or other of the body of the mandible. Where the force of impact is greater, as in most road traffic accidents, the larger indirect force transmitted to the condylar region results in an increase in the number of fractures at this site.

The alveolar resorption which follows tooth loss weakens the mandible and fracture of the edentulous body will result from much smaller impact forces. Extreme alveolar resorption can lead to a situation where, what is in essence a pathological fracture, takes place. Fractures of this nature in a bone perhaps no thicker than a pencil are notoriously difficult to treat.

The teeth

Apart from constituting lines of relative weakness in the lower jaw, the teeth are a potential source of infection of many mandibular fractures. In its physical structure the mandible resembles a long bone, but a long bone which is subjected to a series of compound fractures each time a tooth is extracted. Such an assault on a bone of similar structure such as the femur would lead inevitably to intractable osteomyelitis, whereas in the mandible uneventful healing usually takes place in spite of the wound being bathed in bacteria. The bones of the jaw have developed a special resistance to infection during the course of evolution, the mechanism of which is not really understood.

A fracture of the body of the mandible with a tooth in the fracture line is nevertheless a compound fracture and the tooth, which may have been devitalized, represents a potential source of infection. It is important to take account of this in treating the injury.

Muscle attachments and displacement of fractures

The periosteum is a most important structure in determining the stability or otherwise of a mandibular fracture. The periosteum of the mandible is stout and unyielding and gross displacement of fragments cannot occur if it remains attached to the bone. Periosteum may be stripped from the bone ends by the extremity of the force applied, but frequently it yields to the accumulation of blood seeping from the ruptured cancellous bone. Once the periosteal splint has been removed displacement of the bone ends is free to occur under the influence of the attached muscles.

Fractures at the angle of the mandible

Fractures at the angle of the mandible are influenced by the medial pterygoid–masseter 'sling' of which the medial pterygoid is the stronger component. Fractures in this region have been classified as vertically and horizontally favourable or unfavourable (Figures 2.2 and 2.3). If the vertical direction of the fracture line favours the unopposed action of the medial pterygoid muscle, the posterior fragment will be pulled lingually. If the horizontal direction of the fracture line favours the unopposed action of the

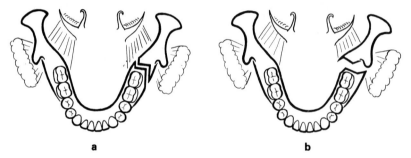

a   **b**

Figure 2.2 a, Vertically favourable fracture at the left angle of the mandible. **b,** Vertically unfavourable fracture at the left angle of the mandible

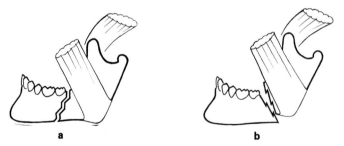

a   **b**

Figure 2.3 a, Horizontally favourable fracture at the angle of the mandible. **b,** Horizontally unfavourable fracture at the angle of the mandible

masseter and medial pterygoid muscle in an upward direction, the posterior fragment will be displaced upwards. It must be remembered that vertically and horizontally unfavourable fractures may be undisplaced if the periosteum is undisturbed. The concept is only important when the periosteum has been ruptured or stripped from the bone. A favourable fracture line will, however, make the reduced fragments easier to stabilize. The presence of an erupted tooth on the posterior fragment will sometimes prevent gross displacement of this fragment in an upward direction if its crown impacts on the opposing upper tooth.

Fractures at the symphysis and parasymphysis

In the symphysis region muscle attachments are also important. The mylohyoid muscle constitutes a diaphragm between the hyoid bone and the mylohyoid ridge on the inner aspect of the mandible. In transverse midline fractures of the symphysis the mylohyoid and geniohyoid muscles act as a stabilizing force (Figure 2.4). An oblique fracture in this region will tend to overlap under the influence of the geniohyoid/mylohyoid diaphragm (Figure 2.5).

When a bilateral parasymphyseal fracture occurs it usually results from considerable force which disrupts the periosteum over a wide area. Such a fracture is readily displaced posteriorly under

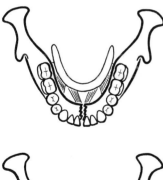

Figure 2.4 Fracture in the midline of the mandible. Minimal displacement occurs in such injuries as the fracture line passes between the genial tubercles

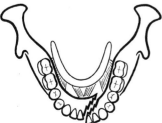

Figure 2.5 Fracture lateral to the midline in the incisor area. The fragment with the genial tubercles is displaced lingually by the pull of the geniohyoid and mylohyoid muscles

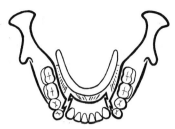

Figure 2.6 Bilateral fracture of the body of the mandible. The anterior fragment is displaced backwards by the pull of the muscles attached to the genial tubercles

the influence of the genioglossus muscle and to a lesser extent the geniohyoid (Figure 2.6). It is often stated that such a fracture removes the attachment of the tongue to the mandible and allows the tongue to fall back and obstruct the oropharynx. This is in fact not the case, as the tongue is still firmly attached to the hyoid bone which in turn remains connected to the mandible by the posterior parts of the mylohyoid muscle. In addition, the intrinsic muscles of the tongue continue to exert control and the tongue remains forward in the oral cavity. Voluntary tongue control is lost only when the patient's level of consciousness is depressed and consequently it is only in these circumstances that the detached symphysis constitutes a threat to the airway.

Fractures of the condylar process

When a fracture of the condylar neck occurs the condylar head is frequently displaced and sometimes dislocates from the articular fossa. The most frequent direction of displacement is medially and forward under the influence of the lateral pterygoid muscle. The importance of this muscle as a displacing force is more dramatically illustrated in those cases where anteromedial dislocation occurs some days after injury in a previously undisplaced fracture.

Fracture of the coronoid process

This is a rare fracture which is said to be brought about by reflex muscular contraction of the strong temporalis muscle which then displaces the fragment upwards towards the infratemporal fossa.

Comminuted fractures

Extensively comminuted fractures, such as occur following missile injuries, may involve a considerable area of mandibular bone.

Where there are strong muscle attachments as at the ramus and angle the amount of displacement of the comminuted segment is often remarkably little. This is explained by the fragmentation at the site of the muscle attachments. The small fragments are pulled away by the contracting muscle leaving the bulk of the comminuted bone relatively undisplaced.

Fractures of the edentulous mandible

Following alveolar resorption the molar areas of the edentulous mandible become much less resistant to fracture. It is not unusual to see bilateral fractures of the body of the edentulous mandible each occurring near the posterior attachment of the mylohyoid diaphragm. The mylohyoid muscle in the edentulous jaw is attached relatively higher up on the lingual side than when the teeth are present. These factors combine to create a situation whereby extreme downward and backward angulation of the anterior part of the mandible takes place under the influence of

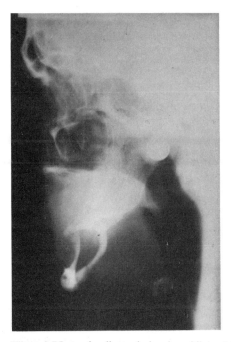

Figure 2.7 Lateral radiograph showing a bilateral fracture of a thin edentulous mandible with a severe 'bucket handle' type of displacement

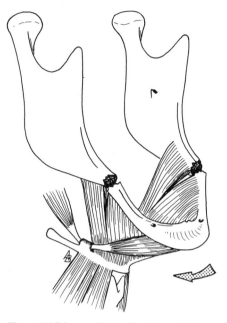

Figure 2.8 Diagram illustrating the probable mechanism producing the type of fracture illustrated in Figure 2.7. The fracture occurs in the resorbed body of the mandible in front of the posterior attachment of the mylohyoid muscle

the digastric and the mylohyoid muscles. This extreme displacement may lead to respiratory distress, particularly in an elderly patient (Seshul *et al.*, 1978). This 'bucket handle' displacement peculiar to the thin edentulous mandible is illustrated in Figures 2.7 and 2.8.

Blood supply of the mandible

An effective blood supply is one of the most important factors in the healing of a fractured bone. The mandible receives an endosteal supply via the inferior dental artery and vein and these vessels are important in young patients. Occasionally a fracture of the body of the mandible will cause a complete rupture of the inferior dental artery. Whereas this vessel usually goes into spasm with spontaneous arrest of haemorrhage, this is not always the case and prolific bleeding can occur which is difficult to control. In these rare emergencies the mandible fracture needs to be reduced immediately by manipulation and the bone ends held in rough alignment by a wire ligature around adjacent teeth.

The other and more important blood supply to the mandible derives from the periosteum. The periosteal supply becomes increasingly important with ageing as the inferior dental artery slowly diminishes in size and eventually disappears (Bradley, 1972). This fact has considerable significance for the healing of fractures in the elderly. Open reduction of fractures in this age group involves elevation of periosteum from the bone ends and further deprivation of blood supply to the fracture site with resultant delayed or non-union.

Other important related anatomical structures

Nerves

The inferior dental nerve is frequently damaged in fractures of the body and angle of the mandible producing anaesthesia or paraesthesia within the distribution of the mental nerve on the side of the injury.

There are numerous reported cases where the facial nerve has been damaged by direct trauma over the mandibular ramus. Facial palsy of the lower motor neurone type results. In certain instances the mandibular condyle may impact with such force against the temporal bone that a fracture of the temporal bone results and in these rare circumstances the facial nerve may be damaged within the fallopian canal (Goin, 1980). Occasionally the mandibular division of the facial nerve is damaged in isolation in association with a fracture of the body or angle.

Blood vessels

Apart from haemorrhage from the inferior dental vessels which has been mentioned, injury to major blood vessels is unusual in association with mandibular fractures.

A large sublingual haematoma may result from rupture of dorsal lingual veins medial to an angle fracture.

The facial vessels are vulnerable to direct trauma where they cross the lower border of the mandible anterior to the angle.

Temporomandibular joint

Traumatic arthritis can occur without a fracture of the condyle, from indirect transmitted violence. A synovial effusion occurs with widening of the joint space on radiographs. Such a joint is extremely painful and mandibular movement very restricted.

When an intracapsular fracture of the condylar head occurs there may be direct involvement of the temporomandibular joint with haemarthrosis. If this occurs in a young child it can lead to fibrous or bony ankylosis of the temporomandibular articulation and destruction of the growth potential of the condyle.

The meniscus is a most important component of the temporomandibular joint. Routine imaging techniques do not delineate this structure and the incidence of meniscal damage in mandibular trauma is not known. Disruption of the meniscus itself or the meniscal attachments may be important as regards the subsequent function of the joint. There is some evidence that tearing of the meniscus along with haemarthrosis predisposes to later fibrous or bony ankylosis (Wheat, Evascus and Laskin, 1977; Laskin, 1978; Yaillen et al., 1979; Bradley, 1985).

Not infrequently a fractured condylar head is driven backwards with sufficient force to tear the adjacent external auditory meatus and cause bleeding from the external ear. Such bleeding must be carefully distinguished from the middle ear bleeding which signifies a fracture of the base of the skull. Very rarely the glenoid fossa is fractured as the mandibular condyle is driven against this thin part of the temporal bone but usually a fracture of the condylar neck prevents the other more serious injury occurring.

Chapter 3

Clinical examination

The examination of a patient with a fracture of the mandible takes place in three stages:

1. Immediate assessment and treatment of any condition constituting a threat to life.
2. General clinical examination of the patient.
3. Local examination of the mandibular fracture.

Immediate assessment

Patients with maxillofacial injuries may have sustained other bodily injury which may constitute an actual threat to life or be of higher priority than the facial trauma. It is therefore always necessary to make a rapid assessment of a newly injured patient and institute any emergency resuscitation before embarking on a more detailed examination. Maxillofacial injury, albeit rarely, threatens the patient's airway and constitutes the highest priority in the treatment schedule. The emergency treatment of mandibular fractures will be considered in more detail in the next chapter.

General clinical examination

Fractures of the mandible are, of course, caused by trauma of varying degrees of severity and it is reasonable to consider the possibility that this degree of trauma may also have caused injury elsewhere in the body. This is especially true if the patient has been involved in a severe accident such as a road traffic accident or a fall from a considerable height. However, a simple blow on the lower jaw as a result of a fight or during the course of some game may result in force being transmitted to the cranium which results in serious injury or even death of the patient. The mere fact that a patient is ambulant and apparently unaffected by the injury does not necessarily preclude the presence of more serious underlying damage.

Killey (1974) described a patient who sustained a simple crack fracture at the angle of the mandible during a game of rugby football. The blow was not sufficient to cause loss of consciousness at the time of the injury and the patient was ambulant when first seen and apparently in good health. Shortly after admission, however, the patient exhibited signs of cerebral haemorrhage, and in spite of neurosurgical intervention, died the following day from a subarachnoid haemorrhage. Similar examples can be quoted from the statistics of fatalities following amateur and professional boxing injuries. It is imperative, therefore, that all traumatic cases should have a careful physical examination and no operative procedure should be carried out to treat a fracture until the operator is certain that the patient has not sustained an additional and more serious injury. Treatment of such an associated condition should, of course, take precedence over the mandibular fracture, but occasionally it may be treated concurrently. It should be remembered that elderly patients may fall and break their mandible as a result of a cerebral or cardiac catastrophe and this possibility must always be considered in such cases.

Fortunately, most major injuries are fairly obvious and careful inspection and gentle palpation of the unclothed body in a good light will usually reveal their presence. It is unusual for a patient with a mandibular fracture to be shocked and if this condition is present some more serious injury should be suspected.

Local examination of the mandibular fracture

Preparation for examination

Prior to a detailed examination of the mandible, the face must be gently cleaned with warm water or swabs to remove caked blood, road dirt, etc. in order that an accurate evaluation of any soft-tissue injury can be made. The mouth, similarly, should be examined for loose or broken teeth or dentures, and any congealed blood removed with swabs held in non-toothed forceps. If a denture is fractured, the fragments should be assembled to make sure that no portion is missing – possibly displaced down the throat. Only after careful cleaning has been carried out both extra- and intra-orally is it possible to evaluate the full extent of the injury.

It is surprising how the magnitude of the surgical problem diminishes as the overlying blood is removed and accurate visualization becomes possible. During this gentle cleaning of the face, the cranium and cervical spine are carefully inspected and then palpated for signs of injury. Finally the mandibular fracture is examined in detail.

Extra-oral examination

Many of the physical signs of a fractured bone result from the extravasation of blood from the damaged bone ends. This results in rapid early swelling from the accumulation of blood within the tissues and later increase in the swelling resulting from increased capillary permeability and oedema. Swelling and ecchymosis indicate the site of any mandibular fracture. There may be obvious deformity in the bony contour of the mandible and if considerable displacement has occurred the patient is unable to close the anterior teeth together and the mouth hangs open. A conscious patient may seek to support the lower jaw with his hand. Many mandibular fractures are compound into the mouth and blood-stained saliva is frequently observed dribbling from the corners of the mouth, particularly if the fracture is recent.

Palpation should begin bilaterally in the condylar region and then continue downwards and along the lower border of the mandible. Bone tenderness is almost pathognomic of a fracture, even an undisplaced crack, but if there is more displacement it may be possible to palpate deformity or elicit bony crepitus.

Fractures of the body of the mandible are often associated with injury to the inferior dental nerve in which case there will be reduced or absent sensation on one or both sides of the lower lip.

Intra-oral examination

It is impossible to assess intra-oral damage if the parts are obscured by blood. Conscious cooperative patients may be given a lukewarm mouthwash but in most cases the clinician will have to remove the clotted blood by gently cleaning the whole area with moistened swabs. Congealed blood and any fragments of teeth, alveolus or dentures are removed carefully by forceps assisted by gentle suction if available.

A good light is essential. The buccal and lingual sulci are examined for ecchymosis. Submucosal extravasation of blood is often indicative of underlying fracture, particularly on the lingual side (Figure 3.1). Ecchymosis in the buccal sulcus is not necessarily the result of a fracture as there is considerable soft tissue overlying the bone in this area and extensive bruising may follow a blow over

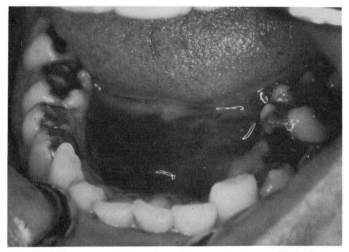

Figure 3.1 Haematoma in floor of mouth as a result of a mandibular fracture

the lower jaw insufficient to cause a fracture. However, on the lingual side the mucosa of the floor of the mouth overlies the periosteum of the mandible which, if breached following a fracture, will invariably be the cause of any leakage of blood into the lingual submucosa. This then is a most valuable sign of bony injury in the body of the mandible. Small linear haematomas, particularly in the third molar region, are reliable indicators of adjacent fracture.

The occlusal plane of the teeth is next examined or, if the patient is edentulous, the alveolar ridge. Step defects in the occlusion or alveolus are noted along with any obvious lacerations of the overlying mucosa. It is important to examine all the individual teeth and to note any luxation or subluxation along with missing crowns, bridges or fillings. Individually fractured teeth must be assessed for involvement of the dentine or pulp. Finally, all teeth should be carefully examined with a mirror and probe to detect loose fillings, fine cracks or splits in the tooth substance. If teeth, portions of teeth, dentures, fillings, etc. are not accounted for, a radiograph of the chest must be ordered in case they have been inhaled.

Possible fracture sites are gently tested for mobility by placing a finger and thumb on each side and using pressure to elicit unnatural mobility. If the patient can cooperate, he is asked to carry out a full range of mandibular movements and any pain or limitation of movement recorded. Occasionally, even this detailed examination fails to confirm a mandibular fracture which is thought to be present from the history and presence of haematoma. In such cases the flat of both hands should be placed over the two angles of the mandible and gentle pressure exerted. This manoeuvre will always elicit pain when even a crack fracture is present, but the procedure should be one of last resort as it produces extreme discomfort if a mobile fracture is present.

Signs and symptoms of mandibular fractures at various fracture sites

Fractures of the mandible can be divided according to their anatomical location into eight main types. These are:

1. Dento-alveolar
2. Condylar
3. Coronoid
4. Ramus
5. Angle
6. Body (molar and premolar areas)
7. Symphysis and parasymphysis
8. Multiple and comminuted fractures.

Fractures in each of these situations have clearly defined signs and symptoms which can be readily elicited even in cases of multiple injury.

Dento-alveolar fractures

Dento-alveolar injuries are defined as those in which avulsion, subluxation or fracture of the teeth occurs in association with a fracture of the alveolus. They may occur alone or in conjunction with some other type of mandibular fracture.

Soft-tissue injuries

Inspection may reveal a full thickness wound of the lower lip or a ragged laceration on its inner aspect caused by impaction against the lower anterior teeth. There is usually substantial bruising of the lips and there may be portions of tooth or foreign bodies embedded in the soft tissues.

Over the alveolar margin itself there will usually be lacerations of the gingiva and deformity of the alveolus. In the anterior region of the mandible a 'degloving' injury may occur as a result of impaction of the point of the chin on some resilient surface such as soft earth. The jaw does not fracture but the soft tissue is rotated violently over the point of the chin and a horizontal tear occurs in the buccal sulcus at the junction of the attached and free gingiva.

Damage to teeth

Fracture of the crown of individual teeth may occur as a direct result of trauma or by forcible impaction against the opposing dentition. Meticulous dental examination is essential and any missing fragments of crown or missing fillings noted. These may be embedded within the soft tissues or more rarely swallowed or inhaled. Exposure or near exposure of the pulp chamber requires immediate treatment if the extent of other injuries permits, and is of greater priority than the immobilization of most associated fractures of the underlying bone.

Fractures of the roots of teeth may be present which are difficult to diagnose clinically. Excessively mobile teeth which do not appear to be subluxed are suspect and should be earmarked for later periapical radiographs. Subluxation of teeth will cause derangement of the occlusion. Individual teeth may be missing and a recent extraction wound suggests that the tooth concerned has been knocked out. Occasionally molar and premolar teeth appear superficially normal but close inspection reveals either a vertical split or a horizontal fracture just below the gingival margin resulting from indirect trauma against the opposing dentition or violent impact by a small hard object such as a missile.

Electrical or thermal vitality tests at this stage of injury are unreliable and of little use in determining the eventual prognosis for the pulp. A blow of sufficient force to disrupt the alveolus will usually disturb the function of the nerve endings supplying individual teeth whose blood supply may nevertheless be intact.

Alveolar fractures

Fractures of the alveolus may be present with or without associated injury to the teeth. However teeth within an alveolar fracture should be presumed to have been devitalized until evidence to the contrary emerges during the period of follow-up. Gross comminution of the alveolus occurs following severe trauma, but more often the alveolar fracture consists of one or two distinct fragments containing teeth (Figures 3.2 and 3.3). A complete alveolar fragment may be displaced into the soft tissues of the floor of the mouth and can on occasions be completely

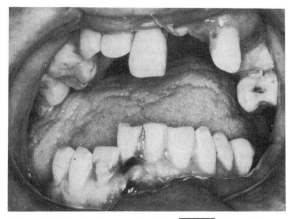

Figure 3.2 Alveolar fracture involving $\overline{1|12345}$. The patient reported to a dental surgeon several days after the injury and insisted that the painful $\overline{3}$ should be extracted. On applying forceps to this tooth the $\overline{1|12345}$ also moved

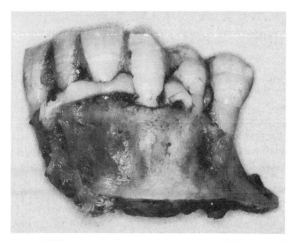

Figure 3.3 The alveolar fracture shown in Figure 3.2 was heavily infected and the fragment had to be removed

covered by mucosa. In the symphysis region it may be difficult to determine whether a loose alveolar fracture is part of a complete fracture of the mandible. An associated fracture through the lower border may be only a crack and less mobile than the alveolar segment. During the initial examination it may be possible gently to reposition loose alveolar fragments and the earlier this is achieved the better the prognosis for individual teeth.

Condylar fractures

These are the most common overall fractures of the mandible and are the ones most commonly missed on clinical examination. Condylar fractures may be unilateral or bilateral and they may either involve the joint compartment as intracapsular fractures or the condylar neck when they are regarded as extracapsular. The latter are the more common. The extracapsular fracture may exist with or without dislocation of the condylar head and the upper fragment may either remain angulated on the lower portion of the ramus or be displaced medially or laterally. The commonest displacement is anteromedial owing to the direction of pull of the lateral pterygoid muscle which is attached to the anteromedial aspect of the condylar head and to the meniscus of the temporomandibular joint.

In the immediate post-traumatic phase most fractures in the condylar region exhibit similar signs and symptoms.

Unilateral condylar fractures

Inspection

There is often swelling over the temporomandibular joint area and there may be haemorrhage from the ear on that side. Bleeding from the ear results from laceration of the anterior wall of the external auditory meatus, caused by violent movement of the condylar head against the skin in this region. In the normal subject the close relationship of the condyle to the skin of the external auditory meatus can be appreciated if the little finger is placed within the external ear and the jaw moved.

It is important to distinguish bleeding originating in the external auditory canal from the more serious middle ear haemorrhage. The latter signifies a fracture of the petrous temporal bone and may be accompanied by cerebrospinal otorrhoea. In all cases of suspected condylar fracture the ear should be examined carefully with an auroscope. The appearance may be extremely confusing even to an experienced maxillofacial surgeon and there should be no hesitation in asking the opinion of an otologist in these circumstances.

The haematoma surrounding a fractured condyle may track downwards and backwards below the external auditory canal. This gives rise to ecchymosis of the skin just below the mastoid process on the same side. This particular physical sign also occurs with fractures of the base of the skull when it is known as 'Battle's sign'.

It is vital not to confuse the aetiology when an ecchymosis at this site is discovered. On the very rare occasion when the condylar head is impacted through the glenoid fossa, the mandible will be locked and middle ear bleeding may present externally. If the condylar head is dislocated medially and all oedema has subsided due to passage of time, it may be possible to observe a characteristic hollow over the region of the condylar head, but in the immediate post-traumatic phase this physical sign is obscured by oedema.

Palpation
In the recently injured patient there is invariably tenderness over the condylar area. When post-traumatic oedema is present it is difficult to palpate the condylar head and what is believed to be the condylar head may, in fact, be that portion of the condylar neck continuous with the lower portion of the ramus. It may be possible to determine whether the condylar head is displaced from the glenoid fossa by palpation within the external auditory meatus. Standing in front of the patient both little fingers can be hooked into each external auditory meatus and the position and movement of each condylar head compared.

Rarely, haemorrhage from the condylar region tracks across the base of the skull and exerts pressure on the mandibular division of

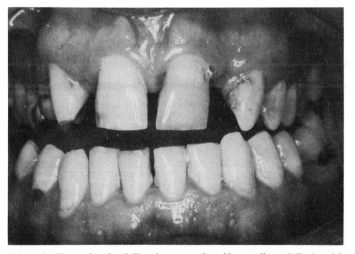

Figure 3.4 Type of occlusal disturbance produced by a unilateral displaced fracture of the condylar neck. The fracture has occurred on the left side with resultant shortening of the ramus and premature contact of the molar teeth

the trigeminal nerve as it emerges from the foramen ovale. This in turn gives rise to paraesthesia of the lower lip in the absence of a fracture of the body or angle of the mandible on that side.

Intra-orally

Displacement of the condyle from the fossa or over-riding of the fractured condylar neck shortens the ramus on that side and produces gagging of the occlusion on the ipsilateral molar teeth (Figure 3.4). The mandible deviates on opening towards the side of the fracture and there is usually painful limitation of protrusion and lateral excursion to the opposite side.

Bilateral condylar fractures

Extra-orally

The signs and symptoms already mentioned for the unilateral fracture may be present on both sides. Overall mandibular movement is usually more restricted than is the case with a unilateral fracture.

Intra-orally

As with the unilateral fracture derangement of the occlusion will be found only if the condyle is displaced on one or other side causing shortening of the ramus. Intracapsular fractures produce little if any shortening and the occlusion is often found to be normal. If both fractures have resulted in displacement of the condyles from the glenoid fossa or over-riding of the fractured bone ends, an anterior open bite is found to be present (Figure 3.5). In all cases of bilateral fracture there is pain and limitation of opening and restricted protrusion and lateral excursions.

Bilateral condylar fractures are frequently associated with fracture of the symphysis or parasymphysis and these areas should always be carefully examined.

Fracture of the coronoid process

This is a rare fracture which is usually considered to result from reflex contracture of the powerful anterior fibres of the temporalis muscle. The fracture can be caused by direct trauma to the ramus but is rarely in isolation in these circumstances. If the tip of the coronoid process is detached, the fragment is pulled upwards towards the infratemporal fossa by the temporalis muscle (see

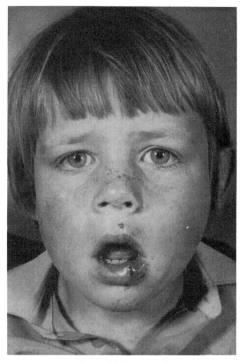

Figure 3.5 A patient with bilateral displaced fractures of the condylar necks. There is an anterior open bite, swelling over both fracture sites and all movements of the lower jaw are restricted

Figure 1.3, p. 7). The coronoid process is sometimes fractured during operations on large cysts of the ramus.

This is a difficult fracture to diagnose clinically but there may be tenderness over the anterior part of the ramus and a tell-tale haematoma. Painful limitation of movement, especially protrusion of the mandible, may be found.

Fracture of the ramus

Fractures confined to the ramus are not common and there are two main types.

1. Single fracture. This is in effect a low condylar fracture with both the coronoid and condylar processes on the upper fragment.

2. Comminuted fracture. Such a fracture always results from direct violence to the side of the face. It is a relatively common fracture in missile injuries but is uncommon in civilian practice. The fragments tend to be splinted between the masseter and medial pterygoid muscles and little displacement occurs unless there has been extreme violence.

Clinical features

Swelling and ecchymosis is usually noted both extra- and intra-orally. There is tenderness over the ramus and movements produce pain over the same area. Severe trismus is usually present.

Fracture of the angle

The signs and symptoms are not markedly influenced by the degree of displacement in these fractures.

Inspection

There is usually swelling at the angle externally and there may be obvious deformity. Within the mouth a step deformity behind the last molar tooth may be visible which is more apparent if no teeth are present in the molar region. Undisplaced fractures are usually revealed by the presence of a small haematoma adjacent to the angle on either the lingual or buccal side or both. Anaesthesia or paraesthesia of the lower lip may be present on the side of the fracture. The occlusion is often deranged.

Palpation

Bone tenderness at the angle externally can always be elicited. Movement or crepitus at the fracture site can be felt if the ramus is steadied between finger and thumb and the body of the mandible moved gently with the other hand. A step may be palpated even if it is not evident on inspection. Movements of the mandible are painful and trismus is usually present to some degree.

Fracture of the body (molar and premolar regions)

The physical signs and symptoms are similar to those of fractures of the angle as far as swelling and bone tenderness are concerned. In the dentate mandible even slight displacement of the fracture causes derangement of the occlusion. Premature contact occurs on the distal fragment because of the displacing action of the muscles attached to the ramus. Because of the firm gingival attachment, fractures between adjacent teeth tend to cause gingival tears. When there is gross displacement, the inferior dental artery may be torn and this can give rise to severe intra-oral haemorrhage. Molar teeth in particular may be split longitudinally in the fracture line and can cause considerable discomfort when the inferior dental nerve remains functional.

Fractures of the parasymphysis and symphysis

These fractures are commonly associated with fractures of one or both condyles. The thickness of the anterior mandible between the canine regions often ensures that these fractures are fine cracks which are little displaced and may be missed if the occlusion is undisturbed locally. The presence of bone tenderness and a small lingual haematoma may be the only physical signs.

Severe impact over the symphysis can lead to considerable disruption of the anatomy. The fracture line is often oblique which allows over-riding of the fragments with lingual inversion of the occlusion on each side. As such fractures are always the result of direct violence there is frequently associated soft-tissue injury of the chin and lower lip.

Such a fracture may often be associated with quite severe concussion, in which case the detachment of the genioglossus

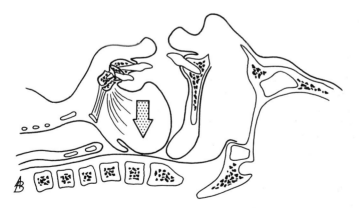

Figure 3.6 Diagrammatic illustration of the mechanism which allows the tongue to fall back and obstruct the airway following a fracture of the symphysis. This is most likely to occur if the patient is unconscious and lying on his back

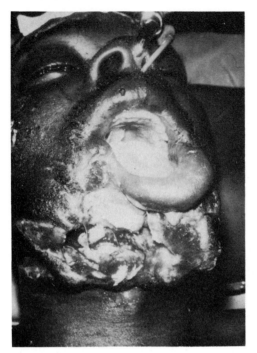

Figure 3.7 Gunshot injury of anterior part of mandible. The patient was not rendered unconscious at the time of injury and had survived 1 week without any airway problems. Under anaesthesia in the supine position control of the tongue is immediately lost and it drops downwards and backwards against the posterior pharyngeal wall

muscle may contribute to loss of tongue control and obstruction of the airway (Figure 3.6). If consciousness is not impaired, considerable disorganization of the anterior mandible and the adjacent soft tissue can take place without any significant loss of voluntary control of the tongue. Direct impact by a small high velocity missile would produce this type of injury without impairment of consciousness (Figures 3.7 and 3.8).

A fracture of the symphysis is not accompanied by anaesthesia of the skin of the mental region unless the mental nerves are injured after emergence from their foramina.

Multiple and comminuted fractures

The physical signs of multiple and comminuted fractures depend on the site and number of the fractures. Multiple and comminuted

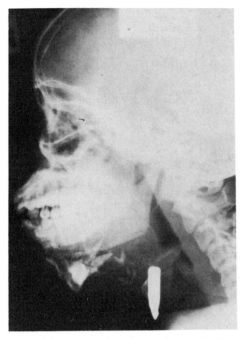

Figure 3.8 Lateral radiograph showing symphysis fracture produced by the bullet which still lies within the tissues. The patient's level of consciousness was not affected by the injury. In spite of the reduced tongue support it can be seen that the shadow of the posterior third of the tongue is postured well forward and the airway is not obstructed

fractures result from extreme direct violence and are usually associated with more severe soft-tissue injury. The precise pattern of bony injury may be impossible to determine from the clinical examination. When there is unexpected mobility of what at first sight appears to be a single fracture, a second fracture on the same side should be suspected. In general comminuted fractures of the ramus, angle and molar regions are not associated with gross displacement of the fragments. However, comminution of the symphysis allows the lateral segments to collapse and presents a much more serious problem of management.

Chapter 4

Radiology

The treatment plan for fractures of the mandible is very dependent on precise radiological diagnosis. It is, for example, most important to know the exact relationship of teeth to a fracture line; to know accurately whether a fracture of the condyle involves the joint space; or to determine the presence or otherwise of comminution of the lower border of the body of the mandible when deciding whether or not to insert a plate or transosseous wire.

Radiographs of the mandible may be divided into essential views which are available in all departments of radiology and desirable views which involve equipment of a more specialized nature. For example, some of the desirable projections are not practical in a severely injured patient who cannot easily be placed in a sitting position. If, however, a skull unit is available these views may be accomplished with the patient lying down.

Essential radiographs

Left and right oblique lateral with the tube angled at 30° towards the lower jaw

This view shows fractures of the body proximal to the canine region, fractures of the angle and fractures of the ramus and condylar regions.

Postero-anterior

The projection demonstrates fractures of the body and angle together with the type of displacement. It is difficult to see the undisplaced condylar head in a normal postero-anterior view as it is obscured by superimposition of the mastoid process. The standard 30° antero-posterior Townes projection demonstrates the condylar region very well along with the posterior fossa of the skull. In order to avoid changing the position of the patient, a *reverse Townes projection* may be used to achieve the same effect. The central ray is angled at 30° to the normal postero-anterior projection which throws the shadow of the condylar head clear of the dense bony structures of the base of the skull.

Rotated postero-anterior

This projection is needed to show fractures between the symphysis and canine regions. To demonstrate this area the head must be rotated from the postero-anterior position until the suspected fracture is in the line of the vertical beam.

Intra-oral

1. Periapical films are required to demonstrate the relationship of teeth to the line of fracture and any damage to the teeth themselves.
2. Occlusal films across the fracture line help to evaluate the relationship of a tooth root to the fracture. They are also invaluable for demonstrating midline fractures of the body of the mandible with minimal displacement.

Desirable radiographs

Panoramic tomography

Equipment for pantomography of the mandible has now become standard in all maxillofacial departments and most patients with mandibular fractures are sufficiently mobile to be placed in the machine. Apparatus has been developed for producing these important diagnostic films in a modified skull unit which allows the radiograph to be taken with the patient lying down.

Pantomograms represent the best single overall view of the mandible and are especially valuable for demonstrating fractures in the condylar region. The combination of a postero-anterior view and a pantomogram obviates the need for further radiographs and significantly reduces the overall radiation dose to the patient (Ching and Hase, 1987).

Standard linear tomography

Precise delineation of a condylar fracture, particularly when the condylar head is displaced, requires tomography, if necessary in two planes. Linear tomography of the temporomandibular joint can be used to demonstrate both the range of movement and the presence or otherwise of intra-articular synovial effusions.

The radiographs should be taken by a radiographer who is experienced in maxillofacial work so as to ensure that the patient is not subjected to unnecessary discomfort.

Computed tomography (CT)

CT axial scans have proved invaluable in the assessment of complex facial trauma especially that of the upper mid-facial region.

They offer very little advantage as a diagnostic tool in the lower third of the face and are not justified for isolated mandibular fractures on either clinical or economic grounds. It should, however, be noted that these sophisticated techniques will demonstrate some details of temporomandibular joint injury, such as a vertical fracture of the condylar head, which are not shown on standard radiographs. If high resolution thin section computed tomography and the presently even more expensive technique of magnetic resonance imaging (MRI) become practical diagnostic investigations in the future, it will be possible to demonstrate the meniscus within the temporomandibular joint and to measure any displacement or damage. This may well have important implications for future treatment of injuries of the craniomandibular articulation (Wilson, 1990).

Chapter 5

Preliminary treatment

The majority of the fractures of the mandible encountered in civilian practice are relatively simple and not associated with other more serious injury elsewhere in the body. It is unusual for such patients to suffer excessive local haemorrhage and evidence of acute circulatory collapse is itself indicative of damage to other important structures. Trauma to the mandible does, however, frequently cause concussion from transmitted violence to the base of the skull.

The airway

Relatively minor injuries which cause intra-oral bleeding and fracture of teeth or dentures can lead to airway obstruction in an unconscious or semi-conscious patient. The essential first aid required consists of careful examination of the mouth and the removal of all fragments of teeth, broken fillings and dentures. If suction is available blood clots and saliva should be evacuated and the patient positioned so that further bleeding and secretions can escape from the oral cavity. If the symphysis region is fractured and particularly if it is comminuted there is some danger of the tongue falling back and obstructing the airway in a patient who has lost voluntary control of the intrinsic musculature. Occasionally a suture passed through the dorsum of the tongue may assist in controlling its position. The most satisfactory posture for an unconscious patient is lying on his side in the position used routinely during recovery from a general anaesthetic. This position should be adopted for transportation of a patient to an accident unit or another treatment centre.

Haemorrhage

Serious haemorrhage is unusual in mandibular fractures. Considerable blood loss can, however, occur when there are extensive associated soft-tissue lacerations. Obvious bleeding points such as the facial vessels should be secured with artery forceps and a temporary dressing applied. Occasionally brisk and persistent haemorrhage originates from a grossly displaced fracture of the body of the mandible. This can only be controlled by manual reduction of the fracture and temporary partial immobilization by means of a suture or wire ligature passed around teeth on each side of the fracture line.

Soft-tissue lacerations

It is desirable to close a soft-tissue wound within 24 hours of injury. As it is often possible to gain access and to stabilize bone fragments through overlying wounds, it is therefore advantageous, where possible, to combine soft-tissue repair with definitive treatment of the fracture. If this is not possible because of the patient's general condition the soft tissues must be dealt with separately under local analgesia as soon as possible after injury. Before closing wounds they must be cleaned to remove foreign material and so avoid subsequent unsightly tattooing of the scar. Wounds should be gently scrubbed if necessary with a mild antiseptic cleanser such as 1% Cetavlon.

Support of the bone fragments

In most cases temporary splinting of the fragments is unnecessary and such devices as the barrel bandage, webbing head cap with chin support, and Elastoplast chin strap are not only superfluous but may in some instances cause the patient additional discomfort. If this type of first aid has been applied it is salutary to observe how often the patient experiences relief when it is removed. Usually if any urgent immobilization of the fragment is required it is best to carry out a definitive standard fixation technique such as an arch bar and not to waste time with an ineffective temporary fixation.

Control of pain

The majority of patients with mandibular fractures do not appear to suffer much pain, perhaps owing to the frequently associated neuropraxia of the inferior dental nerve. Some mobile fractures of the body of the mandible are, however, extremely uncomfortable and a potent cause of restlessness in a cerebrally irritated patient. This situation is one of the rare indications for giving priority to immobilization of the mandible in the presence of other serious injury.

It should be remembered that the use of powerful analgesics such as morphine is contraindicated as they depress the cough reflex and respiratory centre and also mask pain which can be diagnostically important (e.g. from a ruptured spleen).

Control of infection

All fractures of the body of the mandible involving teeth are compound into the mouth and therefore a potential source of infection. Benzylpenicillin should be administered by intramuscular injection of 1 mega unit every 6 hours for the first 2 or 3 days and oral penicillin continued for a further week. In recent years the importance of certain anaerobic organisms in infection of the jaws has been recognized and many clinicians now give parenteral or oral metronidazole 400–800 mg b.d. to all patients with mandibular fractures.

Food and fluid

Food and fluid should, of course, be withheld if an immediate operation under general anaesthesia is contemplated, otherwise fluid may be given as milk and soup using a feeding cup with a spout or tube attachment. A fluid balance chart should be started and kept until such time as the patient is stabilized on a satisfactory fluid intake.

Chapter 6

Fractures of the tooth-bearing section of the mandible

The general principles of treatment of fractures of the mandible do not differ essentially from the treatment of fractures elsewhere in the body. The fragments are reduced into a good position and are then immobilized until such time as bony union occurs. Traditionally immobilization of the mandible has involved linking it temporarily to the opposing jaw by some form of intermaxillary fixation (IMF). This has the considerable disadvantage to the patient of preventing normal jaw function and restricting the diet to a liquid or semi-solid consistency. Weight loss is common, oral hygiene is difficult to maintain and convalescence is prolonged. Leonard (1987) has drawn attention to a thesis by Bruksch at the University of Minnesota in which he demonstrated a 30% reduction of ventilatory volume in patients subjected to inter-maxillary fixation.

For all these reasons, surgeons have looked for alternative methods of treatment which avoided or shortened the period of intermaxillary fixation. The most significant contemporary change in the treatment of mandibular fractures, and in particular fractures of the dentate mandible, has been an increasing trend towards rigid osteosynthesis by means of bone plates. In skilled hands, consistently successful results are now being reported (Cawood, 1985; Prein and Kellman, 1987; Raveh *et al.,* 1987). However, because of the sheer numbers of mandibular fractures and the limitation of resources, such as operating theatre time, a considerable proportion of these fractures will continue to be treated by traditional methods and a general overview is needed in a text such as this.

Reduction

Reduction of a fracture means the restoration of a functional alignment of the bone fragments. In certain situations this does not necessarily imply exact anatomical alignment, e.g. a fracture of the clavicle. However, in the dentate mandible reduction must be anatomically precise when teeth are involved which were previously in good occlusion. Less precise reduction may be acceptable if part of the body of the mandible is edentulous or there are no opposing teeth. The presence of teeth provides an accurate guide in most cases by which the related bony fragments can be aligned. The teeth are used to assist the reduction, check alignment of the fragments and assist in the immobilization. Whenever the occlusion is used as an index of accurate reduction it is important to recognize any pre-existing occlusal abnormalities such as an anterior or lateral open bite. Wear facets on individual teeth can provide valuable clues to previous contact areas. Teeth may on occasions be brought into contact during reduction and yet be occluding incorrectly owing to lingual inclination of the fractured segment.

Widely displaced, multiple or extensively comminuted fractures may be impossible to reduce by means of manipulation of the teeth alone, in which case open operative exploration becomes necessary.

In general, reduction and later immobilization is best effected under general anaesthesia, but occasionally it is possible to employ local analgesia supplemented if necessary by sedation. If there is minimal displacement the reduction can sometimes be effected without an anaesthetic.

If a patient's general medical condition precludes the administration of a general anaesthetic, gradual reduction of fractures can sometimes be carried out by elastic traction. Small elastic bands are applied to cap splints or wires fitted to teeth on the individual mandibular fragments and attached in turn to the intact maxilla. A satisfactory temporary reduction can usually be achieved pending an improvement in the patient's general condition.

Teeth in the fracture line

Teeth in the fracture line are a potential impediment to healing for the following reasons:

1. The fracture is compound into the mouth via the opened periodontal membrane.
2. The tooth may be damaged structurally or lose its blood supply as a result of the trauma so that the pulp subsequently becomes necrotic.
3. The tooth may be affected by some pre-existing pathological process, such as an apical granuloma.

The fracture line can become infected as a result of any of the above; either from the oral cavity via the disrupted periodontium or directly from an infected pulp or apical granuloma. Infection of the fracture line will result in greatly protracted healing of the fracture or even non-union.

For these reasons in pre-antibiotic days all teeth in the line of the fracture were extracted. This practice was, however, continued into the antibiotic era with unnecessary detriment to the patient. A tooth in the line of fracture which is structurally undamaged, potentially functional, and not subluxed should be retained and antibiotics administered. Its retention will tend to delay clinical union of the fracture by a short period, but this is acceptable in order to preserve the integrity of the dentition. Obviously teeth in an intact dentition are more important than those in a partially edentulous jaw.

Without antibiotic therapy teeth in the line of fracture constitute a real risk of infection. As recently as 1978 Neal and co-workers reported a complication rate of 30% in a retrospective study of 207 mandibular fractures, where the average delay in treatment was 3–4 days, and the patients were generally from deprived social backgrounds and uncooperative. Thirty-six infections of the fracture site occurred, the incidence interestingly being unrelated to whether the involved tooth was removed at the time of treatment or after the complications had ensued.

In general the infection rate of mandibular fractures which involve teeth is much lower; around 5% (James et al., 1981). Kahnberg (1979) and Kahnberg and Ridell (1979) in a study of 185 teeth involved in the line of mandibular fractures have shown that the prognosis of the teeth they elected to conserve was good. Complete clinical and radiographic recovery was found in 59%, a figure similar to other studies (Fuhr and Setz, 1963; Roed-Petersen and Andreasen, 1970; Ridell and Astrand, 1971). Careful follow-up of the retained teeth was necessary so that endodontic therapy could be instituted as soon as there were clinical indications. In Kahnberg and Ridell's study 32 of the 185 involved teeth were extracted, 20 of which became necessary after initial fixation of the fracture because of loosening of the teeth or infection of the fracture site.

Considerable controversy exists with regard to functionless third molars involved in mandibular fractures. These teeth are a potential source of infection and, if left, will eventually need to be removed. They have little value in stabilizing the fracture which, if undisplaced, is retained in line by the attached periosteum. Furthermore, such a tooth will never be more easy to remove, because the fracture effectively disimpacts it and as a result it can be elevated with minimal disturbance of bone and periosteum. On balance it would seem more sensible to remove a functionless, potentially troublesome tooth when an operative intervention has become necessary by virtue of the fracture.

Summary

Absolute indications for removal of a tooth from the fracture line:

1. Longitudinal fracture involving the root.
2. Dislocation or subluxation of the tooth from its socket.
3. Presence of periapical infection.
4. Infected fracture line.
5. Acute pericoronitis.

Relative indications for removal of a tooth from the fracture line:

1. Functionless tooth which would eventually be removed electively.
2. Advanced caries.
3. Advanced periodontal disease.
4. Doubtful teeth which could be added to existing dentures.
5. Teeth involved in untreated fractures presenting more than 3 days after injury.

It is desirable that all teeth not covered by these conditions should be retained.

Management of teeth retained in fracture line:

1. Good quality intra-oral periapical radiograph.
2. Institution of appropriate systemic antibiotic therapy.
3. Splinting of tooth if mobile.
4. Endodontic therapy if pulp is exposed.
5. Immediate extraction if fracture becomes infected.
6. Follow-up for 1 year with endodontic therapy if there is demonstrable loss of vitality.

Immobilization

Following accurate reduction of the fragments, the fracture site must be immobilized to allow bone healing to occur. Orthopaedic surgeons have been concerned for some time with the process of fracture healing when either rigid or semi-rigid fixation is employed. The speed of repair of the weight-bearing skeleton is of paramount importance in the eventual rehabilitation of an injured patient. When semi-rigid fixation is used a fracture heals by secondary intention which involves the formation and subsequent organization of callus. This is a relatively slow process and weight bearing must be delayed until full bone replacement has occurred. Even apparently rigid fixation by means of non-compression plating or pinning leaves a gap between the bone ends and bony union requires organization of a primary callus. Key (1932) noted that healing of the arthrodesed knee was accelerated when the opposing bony surfaces were compressed. Later experimental work (Schenk and Willenegger, 1967; Hutzschenreuter *et al.*, 1969; Perren *et al.*, 1969) has confirmed that compression osteosynthesis of both experimental osteotomies and clinical fractures results in primary bone healing without the formation of intermediate callus. This results in more rapid stabilization of the fracture site and much earlier restoration of the mechanical strength of the bone. Reitzik and Schoorl (1983) have compared rigid non-compression osteosynthesis and semi-rigid wired osteosynthesis on either side of the same mandible. Although non-compression plated osteotomies resulted in gap healing with the formation of a small amount of intermediate callus, this was still superior to semi-rigid osteosynthesis with demonstrably increased mechanical strength on the plated side 6 weeks after surgery.

The question arises as to how relevant are these findings to the treatment of mandibular fractures. Unlike a weight-bearing bone, it is only necessary to immobilize the mandible until a stable relationship between the fragments has been achieved. This period is considerably less than would be required for full bony consolidation to take place. Some simple mandibular fractures need no immobilization at all, particularly if a lack of teeth means that precise restoration of the occlusion is not at a premium. Such fractures remain mobile for some time if they are forcibly manipulated but eventually proceed to full bony union. It is indeed difficult to prevent the fractured mandible uniting and malunion is a more frequent complication than non-union.

The overwhelming advantage of rigid fixation is the avoidance of intermaxillary fixation. If that is not possible, bone plates offer no significant gain to the patient either during treatment or in the eventual outcome. In view of the fact that clinical union of mandibular fractures is much quicker than most other bones, compression osteosynthesis must have a very dubious place in any treatment plan.

Period of immobilization

The period of stable fixation required to ensure full restoration of function varies according to the site of fracture, the presence or otherwise of retained teeth in the line of fracture, the age of the patient and the presence or absence of infection. Juniper and Awty (1973) have shown that in favourable circumstances stable clinical union can on average regularly be achieved after 3 weeks at which time fixation can be released.

In fractures of the body of the mandible the blood supply to the fracture site is significant. Where endosteal vascularity is relatively poor as in the ageing jaw, and particularly in the symphysis region, healing tends to be prolonged. In contrast, the rich blood supply and exuberant osteoblastic activity of the child's growing mandible ensures extremely rapid union.

A simple guide to the time of immobilization for fractures of the tooth-bearing area of the lower jaw is as follows:

Young adult
with
Fracture of the angle
receiving   } 3 weeks
Early treatment
in which
Tooth removed from fracture line

If:

(a) Tooth retained in fracture line: add 1 week
(b) Fracture at the symphysis: add 1 week
(c) Age 40 years and over: add 1 or 2 weeks
(d) Children and adolescents: subtract 1 week

Applying this guide it follows that a fracture of the symphysis in a 40-year-old patient where the tooth in the fracture line is retained requires 6 weeks' immobilization (basic 3 weeks + 1 week for less favourable site + 1 week allowed for age + 1 week for tooth retained in the line of fracture).

Rules such as these are designed for guidance only, and it must be emphasized that the fracture must always be tested clinically before the mandible is finally released. The temporary attachments to the dentition should be retained for a further period so that reimmobilization can be carried out if the union of the fracture is found to be inadequate after function has been restored.

Methods of immobilization

(a) Osteosynthesis without intermaxillary fixation:
   (i) Non-compression small plates;
   (ii) Compression plates;
   (iii) Mini-plates;
   (iv) Lag screws.
(b) Intermaxillary fixation:
   (i) Bonded brackets;
   (ii) Dental wiring:
       Direct;
       Eyelet;
   (iii) Arch bars;
   (iv) Cap splints.
(c) Intermaxillary fixation with osteosynthesis:
   (i) Transosseous wiring;
   (ii) Circumferential wiring;
   (iii) External pin fixation;
   (iv) Bone clamps;
   (v) Transfixation with Kirschner wires.

Osteosynthesis without intermaxillary fixation

This can only be achieved by some form of bone plate. Currently three main systems of bone plating are used for fixation of mandibular fractures. Small bone plates based on the Swiss AO system (Arbeitsgemeinschaft für Osteosynthese) and the ASIF technique (Association for the Study of Internal Fixation) are designed for compression (Luhr, 1968; Spiessl, 1972; Becker, 1974; Schilli, 1977; Kai Tu and Tenbulzen, 1985; Pogrel, 1986; Prein and Kellman, 1987; Raveh *et al.*, 1987) but plates of similar dimensions can equally be of simple non-compression design (Figure 6.1). The main alternative which has found favour has been the use of miniaturized plates such as those originally used for injuries to the fingers (Roberts, 1964; Michelet, Deymes and Dessus, 1973; Champy *et al.*, 1978; Cawood, 1985; Wald *et al.*, 1988) (Figure 6.2).

All forms of bone plating provide extremely rigid fixation. However a distinction should be made between semi-rigid plates and compression plates. In the former group a small gap between the bone ends exists which means that a limited amount of primary callus forms, whereas when compression plates are used experimental evidence suggests that primary bone healing takes place without the formation of any intermediate callus. It is

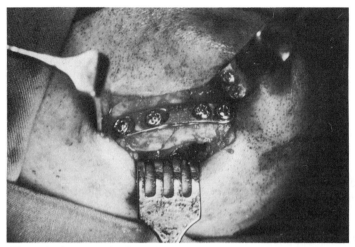

Figure 6.1 A compression bone plate. In this design both of the 'pear' shaped compression holes are to the left of the fracture line. (Case treated by Mr P. T. Blenkinsopp, and reproduced with his kind permission)

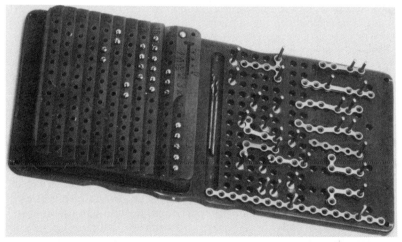

Figure 6.2 A miniaturized plating system based on the original design by Professor M. Champy. (Courtesy of Nagor Ltd, UK)

claimed that the full strength of the bone is thereby restored more rapidly. Each system ensures sufficient rigidity across the fracture site to obviate the need for intermaxillary fixation. This enables the patient to enjoy a relatively normal diet and to maintain oral hygiene more easily. These conditions are desirable for all mandibular fractures but there are particular clinical indications in certain cases. For example, a fracture of the body of the mandible with a coexistent intracapsular fracture of the condyle may make early mobilization especially important in order to ensure recovery of function of the temporomandibular joint. Again intermaxillary fixation is not well tolerated in some elderly patients and is particularly difficult to maintain in mentally disturbed or subnormal individuals.

However, the application of bone plates to the mandible is an exacting technique requiring a fairly long period of general anaesthesia and a considerable degree of surgical skill. Many surgeons routinely still use an extra-oral approach which leaves a scar on the face at the conclusion of treatment. Plating is increasingly carried out from an intra-oral approach (Souyris *et al.*, 1980; Raveh *et al.*, 1987) but the technique requires special surgical instruments in order to gain access to all areas of the body of the mandible.

Becker (1974) has pointed out that any treatment method which does not rely on intermaxillary fixation must ensure the restoration and maintenance of correct occlusion. In spite of numerous claims to the contrary, bone plates because of their very precision do not always achieve this fundamental objective. The occlusal problem can be overcome in skilled hands. Raveh *et al.* (1987) have reported results in 531 mandibular fractures treated with AO plates followed by immediate mobilization. All cases were operated on via an intra-oral approach and only two cases exhibited malocclusion. This group employed a special localization device across the fracture line which was inserted and adjusted prior to the placement of the plate. In other series, however, up to 25% of cases treated required some adjustment by occlusal grinding after bony union was achieved. For this reason a proportion of patients treated by plating techniques are still placed into intermaxillary fixation for a period (Kai Tu and Tenbulzen, 1985; Pogrel, 1986). Plates are particularly useful in patients who are either partially or completely edentulous.

The incidence of postoperative infection of bone plates seems to be decreasing and compares favourably with other methods of fixation. Plating may indeed be employed for the elective treatment of infected fractures (Johansson, Krekmanov and Thomsson, 1988) although the incidence of persistent infection postoperatively is higher than in non-infected cases. Some of these improved results can be attributed to greater surgical skill and some to the use of more biocompatible materials. Titanium is steadily replacing stainless steel and chrome-cobalt alloys for the manufacture of all types of plates. Nevertheless many plates have to be removed due to later infection and in some centres patients are routinely readmitted for elective removal (Battersby, 1967; Souyris *et al.*, 1980).

Non-compression small plates
Small conventional orthopaedic plates have been used in the past for the treatment of mandibular fractures. These plates are, however, larger than the more recently designed mini-plates and offer no advantages (Figure 6.3). The only reason for using a plate of larger dimension than the mini-plates is to incorporate compression across the fracture.

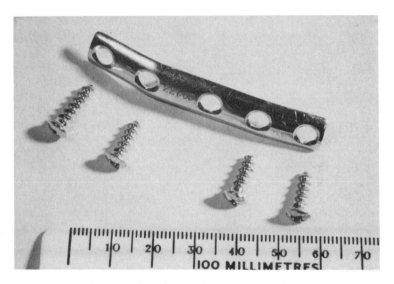

Figure 6.3 A standard non-compression orthopaedic plate which was removed from a treated fracture of the angle of the mandible. Insertion and removal required a large extra-oral submandibular incision

Compression plates
All currently used compression plates are either AO dynamic compression plates or plates based on the same design principle. For anatomical reasons it is necessary to apply these plates to the convex surface of the mandible at its lower border. However skillfully the plate is adapted there is a tendency for the upper border and the lingual plate to open with the final tightening of the

screws. This leads both to distortion of the occlusion and, in a bilateral fracture, to opening of the fracture line on the other side (Spiessl, 1972).

In order to overcome these problems various designs of compression plate have been devised (Spiessl, 1972; Becker, 1974; Schilli, 1977; Prein and Kellman, 1987). Unlike mini-plates (see below) these are often applied to the bone surface using screws which engage the inner cortical plate and must therefore be sited below the inferior dental canal. All compression plates include at least two pear-shaped holes. The widest diameter of the hole lies nearest the fracture line. The screw is inserted in the narrow part of the hole and at the final moment of tightening its head comes to rest in the wider diameter section which is countersunk to receive it (Figure 6.4). The compression holes in the plate may be

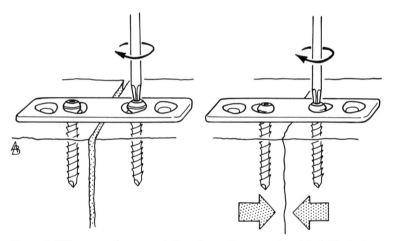

Figure 6.4 Diagrammatic representation of a small compression plate to illustrate the principle by which compression of the bone interface is achieved. The eccentric pear-shaped holes in the plate cause inward movement of the screw at the final stage of tightening when the head of the screw localizes in the wider part of the pear-shaped hole

positioned one on each side of the fracture (Spiessl, 1972) or both on the same side (Becker, 1974). Because of the tendency for the upper border to open when compression is applied across the fracture at the lower border, it is necessary to apply a tension band at the level of the alveolus before tightening the screws (Figures 6.5 and 6.6). This can be in the form of an arch bar ligatured to the teeth or as a separate plate with screws penetrating the outer

A

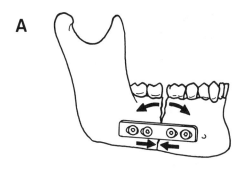

B

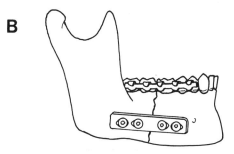

C

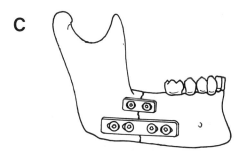

Figure 6.5 Diagram which illustrates the chief problem with a compression plate. **a**, Compression near the lower border opens up the fracture at the alveolar margin. **b**, A tension band previously applied to the teeth prevents the distorting effect of the lower border compression plate. **c**, A similar effect is achieved by prior application of a small cortical non-compression plate above the level of the inferior dental canal

cortex only. Schilli (1977) designed a plate with oblique lateral holes which ensured that the compressing force was in part directed towards the upper border so that when the plate was tightened into place there was less tendency for the fracture line to

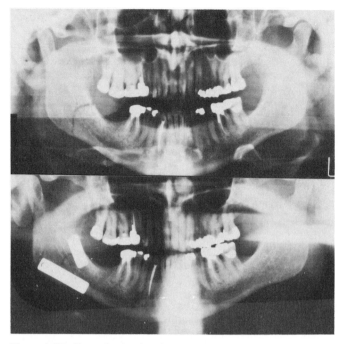

Figure 6.6 Radiographs showing the use of a compression plate at the lower border in conjunction with a non-compression cortical plate above the level of the inferior dental canal. (Case treated by Professor J. Prein and reproduced with his kind permission)

gape. Raveh *et al.* (1987) employed a special adjustable temporary plate at the upper border which enabled them to achieve precise reduction of the fracture prior to application of the definitive lower border dynamic compression plate. They found no application for the eccentric dynamic compression plate in their large series of cases and reported malocclusion post reduction in only 0.5% of patients. Other workers have either placed the patient in temporary intermaxillary fixation or employed special adjustable bone-holding forceps to ensure accurate fracture reduction prior to application of the compression plate.

The operative approach tends to be lengthy and requires considerable expertise to produce consistent results. This is especially so if an intra-oral approach is used or if preliminary intermaxillary fixation is applied. Compression plating becomes more difficult when there is any obliquity of the fracture because of the depth of penetration of the screws. Problems also arise when there is comminution at the lower border which is not always apparent from conventional radiographs. Perhaps the chief disadvantage, however, is the actual bulk volume of the fixation plate which necessitates later removal in a high proportion of patients. This, of course, means subjecting the patient to a further general anaesthetic not otherwise indicated.

Mini-plates

Roberts (1964) used cobalt-chrome alloy metacarpal plates up to 1 inch (2.5 cm) in length to treat a series of mandibular fractures. These were applied to the outer cortical plate after reduction of the fracture, by means of 7 mm long screws 1.5 mm in diameter. Battersby (1967) later reviewed a large series of cases treated in this way and demonstrated satisfactory fixation. The plates were, however, employed as an alternative to transosseous wiring and most patients need to be placed into intermaxillary fixation as well. In 1971 Michelet and Moll described the use of similar small cobalt-chrome alloy plates of various lengths and in 1973 Michelet, Deymes and Dessus reported results in 300 cases. These chrome-cobalt alloy plates were difficult to adapt and were not widely adopted. Champy et al. (1978) introduced a mini-plate system customised for use in mandibular fractures. Originally fashioned in stainless steel, similar plates have now become widely available made from titanium (Figures 6.2, 6.7–6.12).

Champy and his co-workers argued that compression plates were unnecessary because there was a natural line of compression along the lower border of the mandible. They further claimed that compression exerted a stress shielding effect which was detrimental to ultimate mandibular strength. Non-compression mini-plates with screw fixation confined to the outer cortex allow the operator to place plates both immediately sub-apically as well as at the lower border. The stress distribution after fracture of the body of the mandible has been investigated using stressed bars of epoxy resin to simulate the fractured mandible. On the basis of these studies it is suggested that fractures at the angle can be secured with a single plate as near to the upper border as the dental anatomy permits. In the canine region two plates are ideally required, one juxta-alveolar and one at the lower border. All plates can be inserted by an intra-oral approach without the need for intermaxillary fixation (Figures 6.7–6.12).

Mini-plates of this design are now widely used and reported results are encouraging. The operative time involved is no more than required for transosseous wiring. Cawood (1985) has compared 50 cases treated by conventional intermaxillary fixation

54

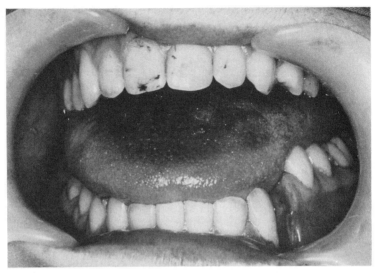

Figure 6.7 The post-traumatic occlusion of a patient with a bilateral fracture of the body of the mandible. The 'step' deformity in the left mandible is clearly illustrated

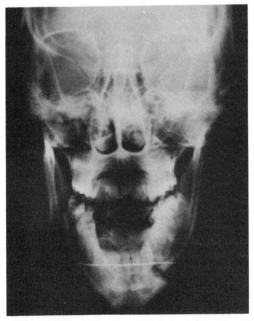

Figure 6.8 Postero-anterior radiograph of the same patient showing fractures in the right molar and left canine regions of the mandible

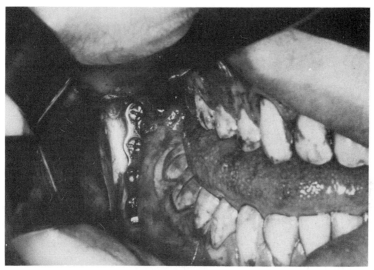

Figure 6.9 Operative photograph of the patient shown in Figures 6.7 and 6.8. A non-compression mini-plate has been applied across the fracture in the right retromolar region

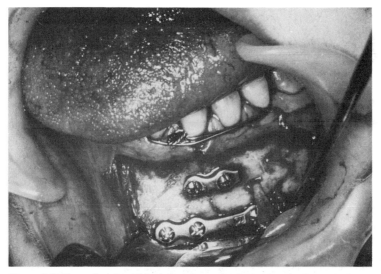

Figure 6.10 Operative view of the left canine region in the same patient as in Figure 6.9. The fracture was reduced with the aid of a temporary wire around the teeth. Two cortical mini-plates have been inserted taking care to avoid damage to the mental nerve which is shown emerging from the mental foramen

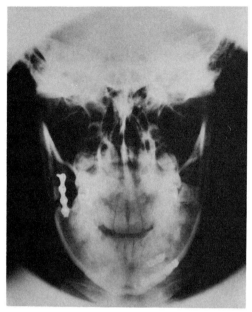

Figure 6.11 Postoperative radiograph of the patient shown in Figures 6.7–6.10. The fractures have been satisfactorily reduced and immobilized by non-compression mini-plates

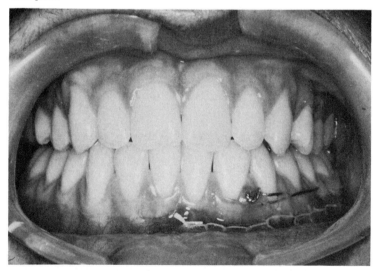

Figure 6.12 Immediate postoperative photograph of the occlusion of the patient shown in Figures 6.7–6.11. The temporary wire ligature round the teeth on each side of the left mandibular body fracture has not yet been removed

with 50 cases treated by mini-plates. The plated series had a higher incidence of residual malocclusion (8%) but there were no cases of delayed union compared with 6% in the control group. Of the plated cases 6% became infected compared with 4% of the controls and 3.8% in a comparable group treated in an independent hospital department.

Postoperative infection of mini-plates appears to vary considerably from unit to unit. Wald *et al.* (1988) have reviewed the literature and report complications as high as 30% in some series. A number of surgeons favour the use of simultaneous intermaxillary fixation when using mini-plates (Mommaerts and Engelke, 1986).

Mini-plate osteosynthesis can be used in virtually all types of mandibular body fracture. Plates can be inserted via an intra-oral approach using special cheek retractors and protective sleeves passed through the soft tissues of the cheek. It is only necessary to reflect periosteum from the outer plate of bone which is an advantage when compared with transosseous wiring. The plates can usually be left in permanently without causing trouble, but on theoretical grounds Cawood (1985) recommends removal because of the continuing effect on the functional forces within the bone.

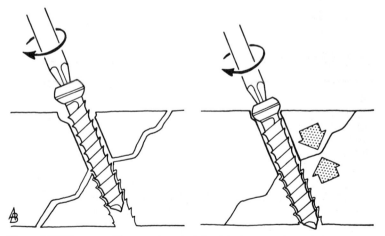

Figure 6.13 Diagram to illustrate the principle of the lag screw in an oblique fracture. The deeper section of the screw hole is accurately tapped whereas the superficial section allows free movement of the screw. As the screw is tightened the fracture is reduced and compressed

Lag screws
A few oblique fractures of the mandible can be rigidly immobilized by inserting two or more screws whose thread engages only the inner plate of bone. The hole drilled in the outer cortex is made to a slightly larger diameter than the threaded part of the screw. When tightened the head of the screw engages in the outer plate and the oblique fracture is compressed. At least two such lag screws are necessary to achieve rigid immobilization (Figure 6.13). The technique has been well reviewed by Leonard (1987) who suggests the technique should also be used when plating an oblique fracture.

Indications for rigid osteosynthesis
Although there are some who would advocate rigid osteosynthesis in all cases of mandibular fracture, there are some fractures which benefit particularly. These are:

1. Fractures in an edentulous part of the body of the mandible.
2. Concomitant fractures of the body and condyle when early mobilization is indicated.
3. Patients in whom intermaxillary fixation is contraindicated.
4. Fractures associated with closed head injury.
5. Continuity defects.
6. Fractures in which non-union or malunion has occurred.

Intermaxillary fixation

In the presence of sufficient numbers of teeth, simple fractures of the tooth-bearing part of the mandible may be adequately immobilized by intermaxillary fixation alone. Clinical union can be expected within 4 weeks in nearly all cases and the fixation can often be applied without resorting to general anaesthesia. A number of methods are available, some of which have proved clinically reliable throughout the history of maxillofacial surgery.

Bonded modified orthodontic brackets
Fractures with minimal displacement in patients with good oral hygiene can be immobilized by bonding a number of modified orthodontic brackets onto the teeth and applying intermaxillary elastic bands (see Figure 9.1, p. 106). The orthodontic brackets can be suitably prepared in the maxillofacial laboratory by welding small hooks onto each of them. Selected teeth in each jaw are then carefully dried, etched, and the brackets bonded to the teeth with composite resin. Because this technique demands complete

elimination of moisture, it is not applicable in cases where there is other than minimal intra-oral bleeding.

Dental wiring
Dental wiring is used when the patient has a complete or almost complete set of suitably shaped teeth. Opinions differ as to the type and gauge of wire used, but 0.45 mm soft stainless steel wire has been found effective. This wire requires stretching before use and should be stretched about 10%. If this is not done the wires become slack after being in position a few days. Care should be taken not to over-stretch the wire as it will become work hardened and brittle.

Numerous techniques have been described for dental wiring, but two have been found very satisfactory. The most simple is direct wiring.

Direct wiring   The middle portion of a 6 inch (15 cm) length of wire is twisted round a suitable tooth and then the free ends are twisted together to produce a 3–4 inch (7.5–10 cm) length of 'plaited' wire. Similar wires are attached to other teeth elsewhere in the upper and lower jaws and then after reduction of the fracture the plaited ends of wires in the upper and lower jaws are

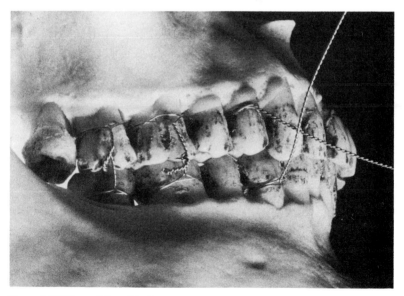

Figure 6.14 Direct wiring of the jaws

in turn twisted together (Figure 6.14). For greater stability the wire surrounding each tooth can be applied in the form of a clove hitch. Thus suitable teeth in the upper and lower jaws are joined together by direct wires.

This is a simple rapid method of immobilizing the jaws, but it has the disadvantage that the intermaxillary wires are connected to the teeth themselves. It is therefore difficult to release the intermaxillary connection without stripping off all the fixation. This disadvantage can be overcome by using interdental eyelet wiring.

Interdental eyelet wiring Eyelets are constructed by holding a 6 inch (15 cm) length of wire by a pair of artery forceps at either end and giving the middle of the wire two turns around a piece of round bar ⅛ inch or 3 mm in diameter which is fixed in an upright position.

These eyelets are fitted between two teeth in the manner shown in Figure 6.15 and twisted tight. Care must be taken to push the wire well down on the lingual and palatal aspect of the teeth before

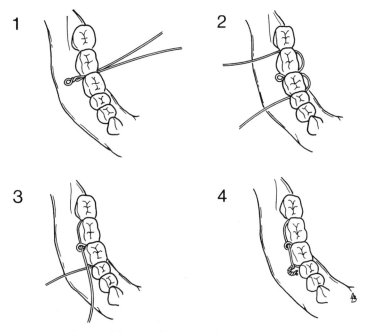

Figure 6.15 Diagram of the stages involved during the insertion of an eyelet wire

twisting the free ends tight, as the eyelet will tend to be displaced up the tooth and become loose. This can be done by pushing the wire down on the lingual and palatal aspects with an instrument such as a flat plastic.

About five eyelets are applied in the upper and five in the lower jaw and then the eyelets are connected with tie wires passing through the eyelets from the upper to the lower jaw. To test whether a fracture is soundly united it is then possible to remove only the tie wires, and if a further period of immobilization is indicated new tie wires can be attached.

The eyelets should be so positioned in the upper and the lower jaw that when the tie wires are threaded through them a cross-bracing effect is achieved (Figure 6.16). If the eyelets are

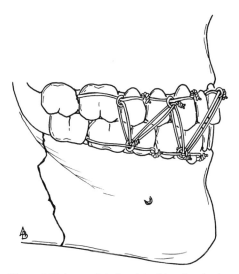

Figure 6.16 A completed eyelet wiring showing how the eyelets are connected by the wires which are twisted in the manner shown in Figure 6.17

placed immediately above each other some mobility of the mandible is possible. It should be remembered when working with wire that the wire is sharp and springy and could readily transfix a patient's eyeball if carelessly handled. Precautions must be taken to protect the eyes at all times and to achieve this object every free end of wire should have a pair of heavy artery forceps attached to it when it is not actually being manipulated. When working under general anaesthesia the eyes should be closed and carefully protected.

After the eyelet wires are fixed the tie wires should be threaded through the eyelets so connecting the eyelets of the upper and lower jaw, but the tie wires are not twisted at this stage. Teeth which require extraction are removed at this time and before completing the intermaxillary fixation the throat pack is removed, after which the fracture is reduced and the tie wire fixation is tightened (Figure 6.17).

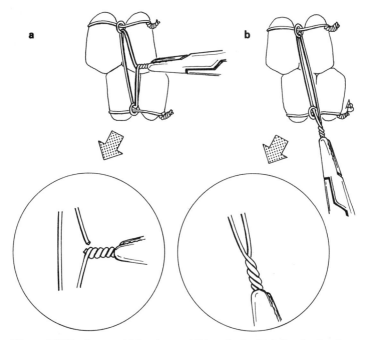

Figure 6.17 The incorrect (**a**) and correct (**b**) methods of twisting the tie wires together. If the twisted portion is at right angles to the wire loop, as shown in **a**, it cannot be twisted tightly without risk of breakage

It is important that the patient's normal pre-fracture occlusion is understood by the operator, for many patients have some abnormality of their occlusion and an attempt to achieve a theoretically correct occlusion in such cases may result in gross derangement of the bony fragments. Much information about the previous occlusion can be inferred from such evidence as wear facets on the teeth, but if the operator is in any doubt about the patient's correct occlusion, study models should be prepared before operation.

Tie wires should be tightened in the molar area, first on one side and then on the other, so working round to the incisor area. It should be remembered that if the wires are tightened on one side first a cross-over bite is produced and if the anterior wires are tightened before the wires in the molar area a posterior open bite results. The wires may be twisted very tight on multirooted teeth, but some caution should be exercised with single-rooted teeth for they may be extracted as a result of force from twisting the tie wire over-tight. It is best to twist the tie wires loosely together first and carry out the final tightening after the occlusion has been checked. Care must be taken to ensure that the tongue is not trapped between the cusps of the teeth. After the interdental eyelet wiring is completed a finger should be run round the patient's mouth to ensure that no loose ends of wire have been left projecting which may ulcerate the soft tissue.

Interdental eyelet wiring is simple to apply and very effective in operation. Excellent reduction and immobilization are effected as the operator can see that the occlusion is perfectly restored. In practice more than half the total number of mandibular fractures can be treated in this fashion.

Arch bars
Arch bars are perhaps the most versatile form of mandibular fixation. They are particularly useful when the patient has an insufficient number of suitably shaped teeth to enable effective interdental eyelet wiring to be carried out or when, in an otherwise intact arch, a direct link across the fracture is required. The method is very simple. The fracture is reduced and then the teeth on the main fragments are tied to a metal bar which has been bent to conform to the dental arch. Many varieties of prefabricated arch bar are available and the Winter, Jelenko and Erich type bars have all proved effective. These bars are supplied in suitable lengths and have hooks or other devices to assist in the maintenance of intermaxillary fixation (Figure 6.18). In the absence of such specialized bars a very effective arch bar can be constructed from ⅛ inch (3 mm) half-round German silver bar. Notches are cut on the bar with the edge of a file to prevent the intermaxillary tie wires from slipping.

Arch bars should be cut to the required length and bent to the correct shape before starting the operation. As the mandibular fragments are displaced owing to the fracture the bar is bent so that it fits around the upper arch. In practice it has been found that such a bar is quite satisfactory when applied to the lower arch as extreme accuracy is not required. When it is impossible to adapt

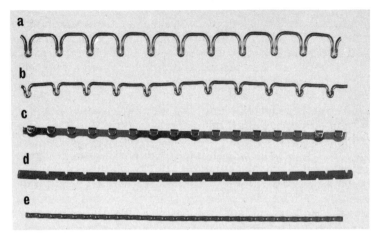

Figure 6.18 Various forms of arch bar in common use. **a** and **b**, Two sizes of Jelenko arch bar. **c**, Érich pattern arch bar. **d** and **e**, Two German silver bars suitably notched to prevent the ligature wires from slipping

the bar to the patient's upper teeth any lower plaster model of approximately the correct size can be used or the bar can be bent to fit another patient with approximately the same size of arch. To facilitate the bending of the German silver bar, it should be annealed by heating it red-hot and then allowing it to cool.

Faced for the first time with the problem of attaching an arch bar to a number of teeth by twisting lengths of 0.45 mm soft stainless steel wire around the teeth and over the bar, any operator would rapidly find a satisfactory solution. In fact, every operator has his own ideal method of achieving this result.

It is helpful after the arch bar has been formed to commence wiring on adjacent teeth preferably in the midline. The arch bar is wired to successive teeth on each side working backwards to each third molar area. In this way minor discrepancies in the arch bar are ironed out as wiring proceeds which produces close adaptation of the bar to the dental arch. The 6 inch (15 cm) lengths of either 0.45 mm or 0.35 mm wire are used for each ligature and some regular pattern is desirable. For instance, each wire may pass over the bar mesially, around the tooth, and under the bar distally, before the ends are twisted together. Whenever contact points between the teeth are tight 0.35 mm wire is used. After all the wires have been placed it will be found that some have become loose and it is therefore important to retighten each wire before the twisted portion is cut and tucked into a position where it will not irritate the tissues (Figure 6.19). Most fractures of the mandible can be effectively treated in this fashion if teeth are present on the main fragments (Figure 6.20).

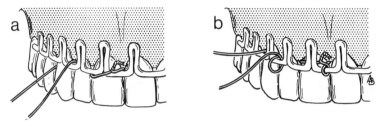

Figure 6.19 Two methods of ligaturing an arch bar to the teeth. **a**, Simple method used in most cases. **b**, Method used for unfavourably shaped teeth allowing the ligature wire to be closely adapted at the cervical margin

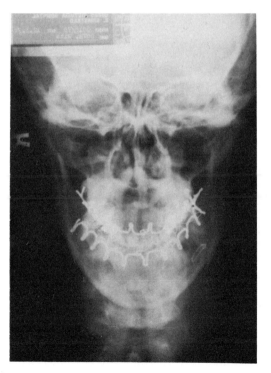

Figure 6.20 Postero-anterior radiograph of a fracture of the left body of the mandible immobilized by arch bars and an upper border transosseous wire

Cap splints

Silver cap splints were for many years the method of choice for the immobilization of all jaw fractures (Figure 6.21). Their present day use in fracture treatment is confined to a small minority of cases. The technique is time consuming both clinically and in the

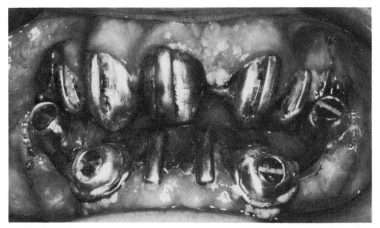

Figure 6.21 Silver-copper alloy cap splints with locking plates and connecting bars used in the treatment of a bilateral fracture of the body of the mandible. The intermaxillary fixation between the hooks has been removed in order to demonstrate the locking plates and connecting bars more clearly

laboratory and the results achieved are accomplished better and faster by other methods. As far as mandibular fractures are concerned, the possible remaining indications for the use of cap splints are as follows:

1. Patients with extensive and advanced periodontal disease when a temporary retention of the dentition is required during the period of fracture healing. A cap splint in this situation will splint all the loose teeth together and allow the application of intermaxillary fixation. Most surgeons would, however, prefer to extract the teeth and apply bone plates to the underlying fracture if the patient was fit for the operative procedure.
2. To provide prolonged fixation on the mandibular teeth in a patient with fractures of the tooth-bearing segment and bilateral displaced fractures of the condylar neck. In such a case the cap splint will immobilize the body fracture and allow mobilization and, if necessary, intermittent elastic traction for the condylar fractures. The cap splint may be built up in the

molar region to provide condylar distraction. Again there are better ways of dealing with this difficult problem (see Chapter 8).

3. Where a portion of the body of the mandible is missing together with substantial soft-tissue loss. A cap splint will allow the remaining tooth-bearing segments to be maintained in their correct relationship pending soft-tissue reconstruction and bone grafting.

Cap splints are still regularly used by some surgeons in orthognathic surgery and they are required for extra-oral fixation in complicated mid-facial fractures, particularly if the mandible is also involved. The method of construction should therefore be understood in principle.

Impression technique   Impressions of the teeth of a patient with a fractured mandible are occasionally needed to facilitate the construction of arch bars as well as for cap splints. The impression technique has to be modified in the injured jaw to take account of limited opening and the presence of blood and excess saliva. The impression need only record the teeth themselves and a small amount of the alveolar margin and it is therefore easier to use a cut back lower impression tray for both jaws. This technique overcomes the problem of decreased opening due to trismus which is usual after fracture of the mandible. Segmental trays are used to take a separate impression of each fragment.

The mouth and teeth must be carefully cleaned to remove as much dried blood as possible. Soft impression materials such as alginate may be difficult to use in these conditions and some operators still prefer to employ composition which can with skill produce an accurate impression of the occlusal surface and permit the construction of a satisfactory cap splint. Such an impression inevitably drags from undercut areas but this can be used to advantage for cap splint manufacture and is no impediment to the making of a suitable preformed arch bar in the maxillofacial laboratory. If the conditions permit, alginate is a more reliable material for the inexperienced operator.

Laboratory instructions   Whatever fixation is proposed, a surgeon will gain useful information from inspection of impressions in the maxillofacial laboratory. He should not leave the design of the splint to the technician but must discuss the case and the surgical plan in detail at the workbench.

Fitting the splint   The completed splints are tried in the mouth before cementation to ensure that they seat accurately onto the occlusal surface of every tooth. Silver alloy cap splints are usually cemented with black copper cement because this material will form a firm bond in the presence of a limited amount of moisture. The material is also a useful obtundent for retained teeth which have exposed and sensitive dentine. Cold-cure acrylic can be used for longer segment splints but the gingival inflammation which occurs after a short period in the mouth is a major disadvantage.

Reduction of the fracture   Cap splints are constructed with small hooks or cleats on the sides to which intermaxillary elastic bands are easily attached. Intermaxillary elastic traction will produce a degree of reduction which may be acceptable in rare circumstances when other injuries discourage prolonged operative treatment of the maxillofacial injury. Operative reduction is to be preferred in all other circumstances. After reduction segmental splints need to be localized together to produce continuity of the splint round the whole mandibular arch. Locking bars have to be made which are soldered to individual plates which in turn can be screwed to matching plates on the splint segments. A completed cap splint is shown in Figure 6.21 and the technique is illustrated in Figures 6.22–6.25.

Intermaxillary fixation with osteosynthesis

Although some simple fractures of the tooth-bearing portion of the mandible can be accurately and adequately treated by intermaxillary fixation alone, in practice that fixation is frequently reinforced by open reduction of the fracture and some type of non-rigid osteosynthesis. Many treatment centres throughout the world do not have access to expensive and specialized systems for applying customised small bone plates and most mandibular fractures are still treated by the combination of intermaxillary fixation and transosseous wiring. There are numerous refinements of these techniques but all have stood the test of time and produce reliable results for the injured patient.

Transosseous wiring
Direct wiring across the fracture line is an effective method of immobilizing fractures of the body of the mandible including the angle. In principle holes are drilled in the bone ends on either side of the fracture line after which a length of 0.45 mm soft stainless steel wire is passed through the holes and across the fracture.

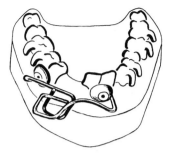

Figure 6.22 Locking plates in position with wire soldered to their outer aspects. These wires are bent over each other, taking care that they do not touch. The plates are then held in position with mounted screws which are not shown on the diagram

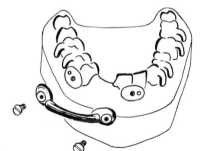

Figure 6.23 Plaster-of-Paris is run over the free ends of the wires and when this is set the locking plates are held in the position they occupy on the splints

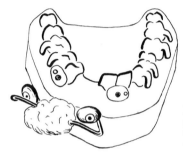

Figure 6.24 A length of ⅛ inch (3 mm) half-round German silver bar is soldered between the inner borders of the opposing locking plates. The wires previously attached to their outer aspects have been cut off

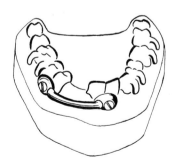

Figure 6.25 Locking plates and connecting bars screwed into position on the splints

After accurate reduction of the fracture the free ends of the wire are twisted tightly, cut off short and the twisted ends tucked into the nearest drill hole. It is most important not to attempt to reduce the fracture by tension on the wire. The fracture must be reduced independently *with the teeth in occlusion* before the wire is tightened (Figure 6.26).

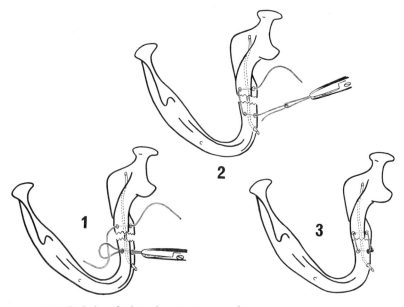

Figure 6.26 Technique for inserting transosseous wires

In practice some ingenuity is required in the placement of transosseous wires in order to ensure that the fracture is stable, particularly when it is comminuted to any degree.

Upper border wires are applied via an intra-oral approach and are particularly useful in aligning an edentulous posterior fragment or for stabilizing a fracture at the angle (Figure 6.27). It is often sufficient for an upper border wire to pass through the outer cortical plate alone as the fixation is always combined with some form of intermaxillary fixation.

Lower border wires are usually inserted via a skin incision placed well below the line of the lower border of the mandible. They are particularly useful for the control of grossly displaced fractures of the body or angle particularly when the upper alveolar border is comminuted. In the symphysis region a lower border

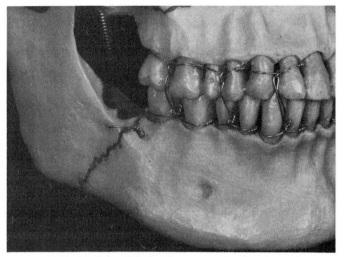

Figure 6.27 Model of mandible showing an upper border wire used to control a horizontally unfavourable fracture of the angle after removal of the third molar involved in the line of the fracture

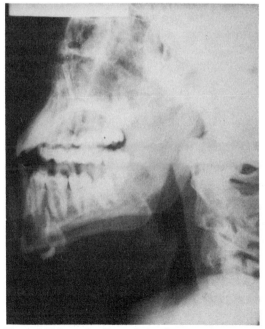

Figure 6.28 Lateral radiograph showing extensive comminution of the symphysis and parasymphyseal region of the mandible together with a fracture of the middle third

wire can be inserted quite easily via an intra-oral incision in the anterior buccal sulcus. Fractures in this area tend to gape at the lower border under the influence of the mylohyoid diaphragm and a transosseous wire placed near the lower border exerts excellent control even when passed through the outer cortex alone.

Multiple fractures at the symphysis create a particularly difficult problem especially when the lower anterior teeth are damaged beyond repair. In such cases the only reasonably large fragments may be those which previously constituted the lower border. Careful multiple transosseous wiring through a submental incision will allow the lower border to be reconstituted accurately, and provide a firm base for restoration of the mandibular arch (Figures 6.28 and 6.29).

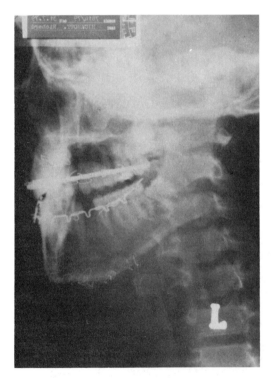

Figure 6.29 Rotated postero-anterior view of the symphysis region to show the multiple lower border transosseous wires employed to restore the contour. (The radiograph has been taken after clinical union when the intermaxillary fixation had been removed)

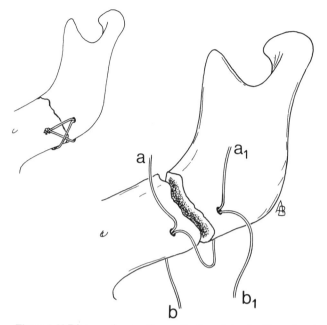

Figure 6.30 Diagram showing the application of standard lower border transosseous wire together with a figure-of-eight wire

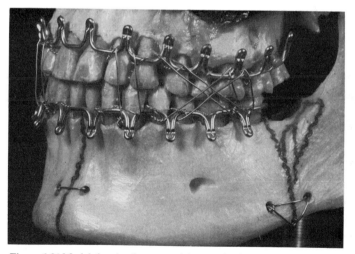

Figure 6.31 Model showing fractures of the symphysis and left angle. A cortical transosseous wire has been placed across the symphyseal fracture and two lower border wires have been used at the angle as in Figure 6.30. The arch bars are Jelenko pattern

When a single lower border wire is applied to a fracture site it may on its own be insufficient to stabilize the fracture owing to the tendency of the fragments to over-ride, particularly if the fracture line is oblique. This can be corrected to some extent by combining a conventional wire with a second figure-of-eight wire (Figures 6.30 and 6.31). Alternatively, the transosseous wire can be reinforced by passing it through a length of stainless steel orthodontic tubing let into a groove in the outer cortical plate (Figures 6.32 and 6.33).

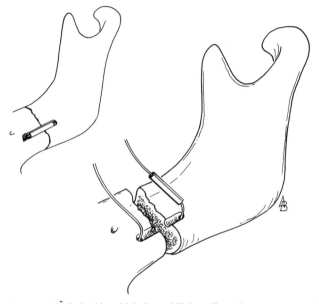

Figure 6.32 Method by which the stabilizing effect of a transosseous wire can be enhanced by employing a length of stainless steel orthodontic tubing let into a prepared groove in the outer cortical plate

When the line of the fracture is very oblique in the vertical plane it is often possible to hold the fracture in a reduced position and pass two wires separately directly through the outer and inner cortical plate and twist the ends together under the lower border, a technique which provides very rigid fixation (Figure 6.34).

Infection of a fracture line prior to definitive treatment has traditionally been regarded as a contraindication to any form of direct skeletal fixation. Indeed at one time it was considered inadvisable to insert a transosseous wire if the fracture was compound into the mouth, because of the risk of subsequent

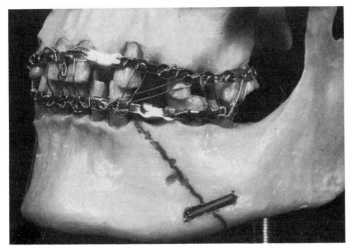

Figure 6.33 Model showing reinforced transosseous wire applied at the angle of the mandible by the method illustrated in Figure 6.32. The arch bars attached to the teeth are Erich pattern

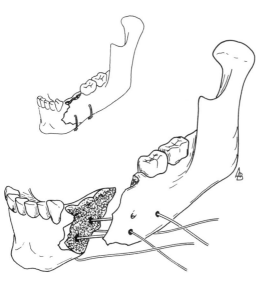

Figure 6.34 Method of immobilizing an oblique fracture by two transosseous wires passed from buccal to lingual and twisted together under the lower border

infection. However, with the routine employment of prophylactic antibiotic cover, this risk is very considerably reduced. James, Fredrickson and Kent (1981) in a prospective study of 422 mandibular fractures concluded that the postoperative infection rate of the fracture line was no different whether closed or open techniques were employed. There is some evidence that rigid fixation of previously infected fractures by plates produces better results regarding uncomplicated healing than traditional methods (Kai Tu and Tenbulzen, 1985). Awty and Banks (1971) and Banks (1985) showed that transosseous wiring could be regularly and safely employed in heavily contaminated gun shot wounds.

Osteosynthesis by wiring has the advantage that minimal specialized equipment is required, and the method can be used to treat most mandibular fractures which cannot satisfactorily be managed by eyelet or arch wiring alone.

Circumferential wiring
A few oblique fractures of the body of the mandible can be reinforced by passing a length of 0.45 mm soft stainless steel wire circumferentially utilizing the same technique as that employed for wiring modified Gunning-type splints to the edentulous jaw (see Chapter 7). A useful variation of this technique is frequently applicable to oblique fractures of the angle after removal of an involved third molar. The wire is passed through the upper border of the proximal fragment and then around the lower border of the mandible which, in an oblique fracture of this nature, controls the distal fragment.

External pin fixation
There are occasions when extensive comminution of the whole or a large part of the body of the mandible occurs. In order to maintain the relationship of the major fragments some form of external pin fixation can often usefully be applied. The technique consists of inserting into each major bone fragment a pair of ⅛ inch (3 mm) titanium or stainless steel pins which diverge from each other, but are connected by a cross bar which is attached to each pin by means of universal joints. Self-tapping pins such as Moule or Toller type are used, these being screwed into prepared holes in the bone of slightly smaller diameter. After reduction of the fracture the pairs of pins are linked by attaching a connecting rod or rods to the centre of the cross-bar by means of universal joints. Alternatively, one end of the linkage may be attached to a lower cap splint by a suitably designed locking plate and connecting bar.

Pin fixation of this nature is not particularly rigid and supplementary intermaxillary fixation is usually required. The extra-oral fixation can be reinforced by self-curing acrylic resin as a biphasic appliance (Morris, 1949; Wessberg *et al.*, 1979). This form of fixation has been widely favoured for the management of missile injuries of the mandible (Kersten and McQuarrie, 1975).

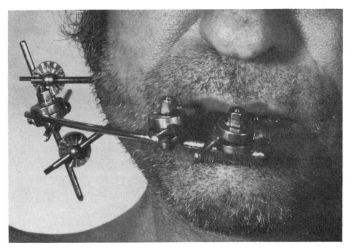

Figure 6.35 Use of bone pins, rods and universal joints to provide extra-oral fixation across an infected fracture at the right angle of the mandible. The connecting bars at the front are attached to a silver cap splint on the lower dental arch

The main indications for the use of pin fixation for mandibular fractures may be summarized as follows:

1. To provide fixation across an infected fracture line (Figure 6.35).
2. To maintain the relative position of major fragments in extensively comminuted fractures.
3. In the treatment of bimaxillary fractures when a 'box frame' form of fixation is employed.

Bone clamps
Another form of external fixation for mandibular fractures utilizes bone clamps. The Brenthurst splint is the best known example of this system. Instead of pins screwed into the bone, the fragments each side of the fracture are secured by clamps attached to the

lower border of the mandible. Pins which project from the clamps are then connected by a system of external rods and universal joints in a similar manner to that employed with external pin fixation.

Bone clamps were introduced to overcome some of the problems associated with the stainless steel bone pins in use at the time. These problems arose from the electrolytic activity produced by biologically incompatible alloys. Since the introduction of titanium these problems no longer exist and as a result bone clamp systems are rarely, if ever, employed for fractures of the tooth-bearing portion of the mandible.

Transfixation with Kirschner wires
Kirschner wires (K-wires) are widely used in orthopaedic practice and are therefore usually available in most hospitals. In rare emergency situations these wires can be used to provide temporary stabilization of a fractured mandible. The fracture is held in a reduced position and one or more wires drilled through the fragments so that part of the wire passes through undamaged bone each side of the fracture. The method is versatile and can be applied with appropriate ingenuity to fractures in any part of the mandible whether there be teeth present or not (Vero, 1968). In the context of fractures of the tooth-bearing area it is of little use when more conventional methods are available.

Shuker (1985) has recently described an ingenious use of a single K-wire for the rapid immobilization of a comminuted fracture of the body of the mandible such as might occur after a missile injury. A horseshoe-shaped 2 mm K-wire is adapted to the mandibular arch and then each end is inserted into two holes drilled from an intra-oral approach into the anterior border of each ramus. The horseshoe-shaped wire lies on the buccal side of the displaced mandibular arch and the individual segments with their contained teeth are ligatured to this semi-rigid frame.

Choice of method of immobilization

A number of interrelated factors determine the choice of a method of treatment. Some of these may be enumerated as follows:

1. The fracture pattern.
2. The skill of the operator.
3. The resources available.
4. The general medical condition of the patient.

5. The presence of other injuries.
6. The degree of local contamination and infection.
7. Associated soft-tissue injury or loss.

The simplest method of treatment is not necessarily synonymous with the best and maxillofacial surgeons need to be trained in all available skills to best serve the patient under their care. Increasingly direct skeletal fixation without the need for total immobilization of the jaw is being shown to produce consistently good results. Such methods demand special skills and resources to match. Even with special skills the necessary surgical instrumentation may not be available. The most complicated of fractures of the mandible can be successfully treated with a suitable selection of arch bars and 0.45 mm soft stainless steel wire and these traditional techniques should not be lightly discarded. It should be remembered that in fractures of the tooth-bearing portion of the mandible the restoration of the occlusion is of prime concern and methods which rely at least in part on intermaxillary fixation consistently achieve this end.

Cap splints have almost been superseded by other methods but the maxillofacial technician remains an essential part of the treatment team, and in particular in the field of reconstruction.

Often more than one technique would be suitable and the eventual choice may depend on such factors as the general condition of the patient, the timing of the treatment of other injuries, the presence of infection and even the availability of an operating theatre.

Chapter 7

Fractures of the edentulous mandible

Introduction

The physical characteristics of the body of the mandible are altered considerably following the loss of the teeth. In effect from the point of view of treatment, the edentulous mandible becomes a different bone. Following resorption of the alveolar process, the vertical depth of the subsequent denture-bearing area is reduced by approximately one-half and in some cases by considerably more. The resistance of the bone to trauma is further reduced by changes in the structure of the bone associated with the process of ageing.

The ageing process is also associated with significant changes in the vascular architecture (Cohen, 1960; Bradley, 1975). The endosteal blood supply from the inferior dental vessels begins to disappear and the bone becomes increasingly dependent on the periosteal network of vessels.

The denture-bearing area of the edentulous mandible is therefore not only more easily fractured, but also less well disposed to rapid and uneventful healing.

In addition, the smaller cross-sectional area of bone at the fracture site and the absence of the stabilizing influence of teeth means that the bone ends are more easily displaced, and even after reduction the area of contact between them may be insufficient for healing to occur easily. The more atrophic the mandible the more significant these factors become and Bruce and Strachen (1976), in a study of 146 fractures occurring in thin mandibles treated by a variety of methods, reported a 20% incidence of non-union.

The edentulous state confers a few advantages. Fractures are, for instance, much less frequently compound into the mouth than when teeth are present. As a result whenever closed reduction is possible the risk of subsequent infection of the fracture is negligible (Amaratunga, 1988). Again the absence of teeth means that precise reduction, such as would be required to restore the occlusion of natural teeth, is not necessary as any inaccuracy is easily compensated by adjustment of dentures. For these reasons many fractures in edentulous patients require no treatment at all. If the fracture is simple with little or no displacement it will heal satisfactorily if the patient refrains from unnecessary active movements and adjusts to a temporary soft diet. Any subsequent discrepancy in the denture occlusion can be corrected in most cases by relining with or without occlusal adjustment.

Reduction

For the reasons already stated, precise anatomical reduction is not necessary in fractures of the denture-bearing area. This is fortunate because reduction is frequently difficult when there is over-riding of the bone ends. Reduction and subsequent fixation become more difficult as the mandible atrophies. The dilemma which often faces the clinician has been well summarized by Marciani and Hill (1979). The reduced cross-section of bone fractures of thin mandibles means that displacement occurs more readily and in this situation open reduction may be the only way to restore adequate bone contact. However, operative open reduction involves further disruption of the periosteal attachment which interferes significantly with postoperative repair of bone. Mature clinical judgement is required, the objective being to achieve sufficient bone contact and alignment with the minimum direct operative interference at the fracture site.

Methods of immobilization

The fact that there is no uniformly accepted method of immobilizing edentulous fractures is indicative of the fact that no completely satisfactory method has yet been devised. There is no doubt, however, that the traditional treatment by means of Gunning-type splints has been largely superseded in recent years by methods which employ some form of direct or indirect skeletal fixation. In older patients intermaxillary fixation is even less desirable than in younger age groups. Nutritional requirements become difficult to maintain and oral candidiasis commonly affects the oral mucosa causing considerable discomfort during the active treatment period. The methods of treatment currently in common use are:

1. Direct osteosynthesis:
   (a) Bone plates
   (b) Transosseous wiring

(c) Circumferential wiring or straps
(d) Transfixation with Kirschner wires
(e) Fixation using cortico-cancellous bone graft.
2. Indirect skeletal fixation:
   (a) Pin fixation
   (b) Bone clamps.
3. Intermaxillary fixation using Gunning-type splints:
   (a) Used alone
   (b) Combined with other methods.

Direct osteosynthesis

Bone plates

Bone plates are particularly useful for displaced fractures of the edentulous mandible, particularly those at the angle. They allow the fracture to be stabilized without immobilization of the jaw as a whole. The patient is, as a result, more comfortable during the period of healing of the fracture. The main mandibular plating systems described in Chapter 6 are in general applicable to edentulous fractures. The reduced depth of bone in the edentulous mandible favours the use of non-compression mini-plates rather than the bulkier compression plates in that the former are less likely to interfere with the edge of a future denture. Bone plates are easier to apply in the edentulous state than when teeth are present as there is no need to achieve the same degree of precision in the reduction of the fracture. Any discrepancy in the eventual occlusion of the pre-existing dentures is more easily corrected than when natural teeth are involved (Figure 7.1).

The surgical technique is, however, more time consuming and requires liberal exposure of the fracture site with extensive elevation of the periosteum. Both compression and non-compression systems require an adequate blood supply to achieve uncomplicated bony union (Rhinelander, 1974) and elevation of periosteum in the thinner mandible seriously compromises the blood supply to the fracture site. It has been suggested that in these circumstances plates should be applied with an intervening layer of attached periosteum (Bradley, 1975), but in practice this is difficult to accomplish.

Plates related to the denture-bearing part of the mandible are much more likely to require removal at a later date than those used in the ramus or in dentate fracture sites. Nevertheless they are currently the preferred method of fixation for the majority of edentulous mandibular body fractures.

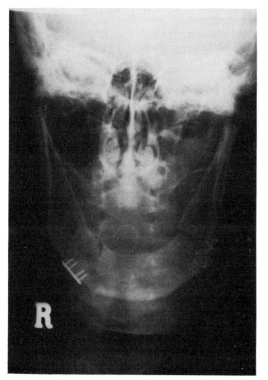

Figure 7.1 Postero-anterior radiograph of a bilateral fracture of an edentulous mandible. A small titanium mandibular bone plane has been applied at the right angle and two transosseous lower border wires at the left angle. No intermaxillary fixation was employed in this case

Transosseous wiring

Many simple edentulous fractures can be satisfactorily immobilized by direct transosseous wires but, in general, when a surgical exposure has been made it is just as easy to apply a mini-plate if available. Transosseous wires do not provide rigid osteosynthesis and supplementary fixation may be necessary. They are somewhat easier to apply from an intra-oral approach and, when placed near the upper border, are less likely to impinge on denture flanges at a later date. In general less periosteal stripping is required on each side of the fracture which may be advantageous when dealing with a very thin mandible. When the neurovascular bundle crosses the fracture site it is easier to avoid damage with a transosseous wire than a screwed plate.

The special instrumentation required for the application of miniaturized plates is not universally available in all parts of the world where fractures require treatment and wiring techniques continue to provide a simple and reliable alternative.

Circumferential wiring or straps

Oblique fractures of the edentulous mandible can be most effectively and simply immobilized by circumferential wires. A modification of the method illustrated in Figure 6.34 is recommended in order to avoid placing the upper part of the wire immediately below the oral mucosa. Williams (1985) has described the use of miniaturized circumferential nylon straps as a useful alternative to wire.

Transfixation with Kirschner wires

This method of fixation employs a 2 mm Kirschner wire inserted within the medullary cavity across the fracture site. When the edentulous mandible is reasonably thick the wire can be introduced through a stab incision in the overlying skin and a suitable point of insertion located on the cortex of the distal fragment. A hole is drilled through the cortex at this point and the wire directed into the medullary cavity and onwards across the reduced fracture site. The wire is cut off at the skin entry point from where it can be withdrawn when the fracture has healed.

In practice it is extremely difficult to insert a wire in this way without damaging the inferior dental vessels and nerve. The most satisfactory method of placing such a wire is to expose the fracture site by an external skin incision. The transfixing wire is passed first into the proximal or distal segment and drilled down the centre of the mandible to emerge through the cortex and skin at a point where the curvature of the jaw prevents further passage. The wire end attached to the drill will eventually come to lie opposite the fracture site at which point the inserting drill is detached and the direction of the wire reversed so that it is made to pass back down the other fragment transfixing the fracture (McDowell et al., 1954; Vero, 1968).

When the wire is inserted under direct vision, as in this latter technique, it can be usefully employed to immobilize fractures of the body of thin edentulous mandibles where a plate would be too bulky (Figure 7.2). It is not possible, however, to employ the technique in the ultra-thin mandible because of the risk of damage to the inferior dental nerve.

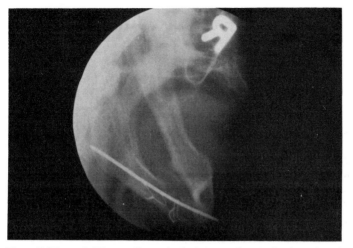

Figure 7.2 Lateral oblique radiograph of a fracture of the body of an edentulous mandible. The transosseous wires alone provided insufficient fixation. The mandible is sufficiently thick to allow a Kirschner wire to be inserted for additional stability without damaging the inferior dental nerve

Primary bone grafting

In 1973 Obwegeser and Sailer suggested primary bone grafting as a method of stabilizing and augmenting a fracture of the body of the ultra-thin edentulous mandible. Wood *et al.* (1979) successfully treated nine such fractures using autogenous rib grafts. A 5 cm length of rib is obtained as an autogenous graft. The rib is split and the two pieces are placed one on each side of the fracture site in the manner of a first-aid splint applied to a limb. The rib halves are lashed together by a series of circumferential wires sandwiching the fractured bone ends between them. Iliac bone can be employed in a similar fashion (James, 1976). Postoperative morbidity at the donor site can be considerably reduced by controlled infusion of bupivacaine through an epidural catheter.

Although the technique appears demanding for an elderly patient it is in practice often less time consuming than bone plating and does offer an effective remedy for what is without doubt the most difficult of all jaw fractures (Figures 7.3 and 7.4).

Indirect skeletal fixation

A system of bone pins joined together by rods and universal joints can be used in edentulous mandibular fractures in the same

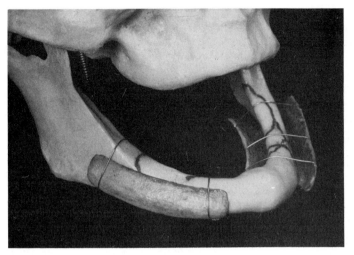

Figure 7.3 Model of edentulous mandible showing how a split-rib bone graft can be applied. In practice more than three circumferential wires are usually employed at each site

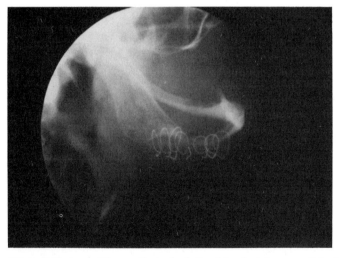

Figure 7.4 Lateral oblique radiograph of ultra-thin edentulous mandible. A split-rib bone graft has been used to immobilize the fracture of the body of the mandible. Stable union was present after 6 weeks

manner as when teeth are present. The method is occasionally of practical use when there has been extensive comminution of a long segment particularly if this involves the symphysis.

Bone clamps such as the Brenthurst splint are theoretically of use to immobilize a fracture in a thin edentulous mandible avoiding direct surgical exposure of the fracture site. In view of the reported high incidence of non-union following open reduction of fractures of the atrophic mandible (Marciani and Hill, 1979), there would seem to be some merit in exploring the clinical usefulness of this method of fixation in the future.

Intermaxillary fixation using Gunning-type splints

The dental splint described originally by Gunning in 1866 was a vulcanite overlay of the natural teeth which he used as a splint for the fractured dentate mandible. A similar splint for the edentulous mandible consisted of a type of removable monobloc resembling two bite blocks joined together. The modern Gunning splint is therefore more correctly described as a Gunning-type splint. These splints take the form of modified dentures with bite blocks in place of the molar teeth and a space in the incisor area to facilitate feeding (Figures 7.5 and 7.6). They can be used when the patient is edentulous in one or both jaws. If the patient is completely edentulous immobilization is carried out by attaching the upper splint to the maxilla by peralveolar wires and the lower

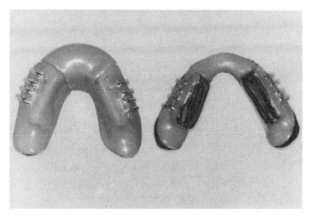

Figure 7.5 Gunning-type splints. The lower splint on the right has a trough on its upper surface filled with gutta percha into which the upper splint fits. This enables the vertical dimension of the bite to be adjusted

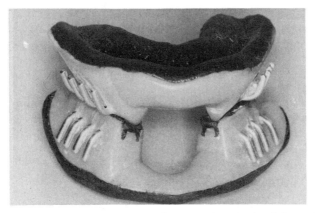

Figure 7.6 Upper and lower Gunning-type splints showing fitting surface of splints lined with gutta percha

splint to the mandibular body by circumferential wires. Intermaxillary fixation can then be effected by connecting the two splints with wire loops or elastic bands (Figure 7.7). When the patient is edentulous in one jaw intermaxillary fixation is achieved by attaching the Gunning splint to whatever type of splint is present in the opposing jaw.

Properly constructed Gunning-type splints should hold the jaws in a slightly over-closed relationship, as in this position fractures of

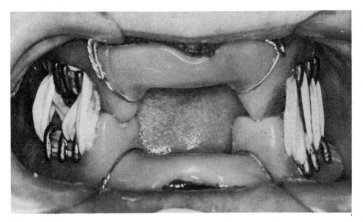

Figure 7.7 Gunning-type splints showing circumferential and peralveolar wires in position. Intermaxillary fixation is effected with elastic bands between the upper and lower hooks

the body of the mandible are more effectively reduced. The edges of the splints should be slightly over-extended around the sulcus in order to minimize food entry under the fitting surface. When the jaws are immobilized over-extension does not lead to ulceration of the mucosa as it would in a functioning denture.

Whenever possible the splints should be constructed on models from impressions of the patient's mouth. The necessary degree of over-extension of the sulcus is achieved by using composition as an impression material which is superior to other impression materials for this one purpose. It is, however, difficult to take an adequate impression when the mandible is badly fractured and the alveolar ridge distorted by displacement of the fragments. It may be possible to make use of the patient's dentures if they are available but it should be stressed that models constructed from the fitting surface of dentures are usually inaccurate and under-extended (Figure 7.8).

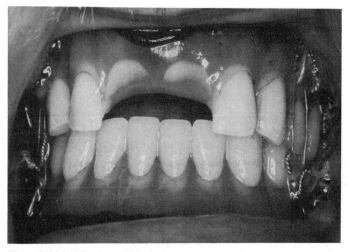

Figure 7.8 Modification of the patient's dentures to form a Gunning-type splint. Hooks have been attached to the dentures on each side by means of self-curing acrylic resin. Wire loops have been used in this case for intermaxillary fixation

The splints are constructed in acrylic resin and the fitting surface is lined with black gutta percha. If the correct vertical dimension of the bite is known or has been recorded the occluding surfaces can be made to fit together satisfactorily in a slightly over-closed relationship. Alternatively a trough can be cut in the occlusal surface of one splint and filled with gutta percha. The opposing occlusal surface is then shaped to fit into the trough and a satisfactory fit obtained at operation by softening the gutta percha and pressing the two splints together (Figures 7.5 and 7.6). Hooks are incorporated into each splint to allow intermaxillary fixation to be applied.

When the facilities of a maxillofacial laboratory are not easily available, splints can be made by modification of the patient's dentures if these have been preserved. The fitting surface is ground away to an even depth and replaced by a liberal lining of black gutta percha. The anterior teeth are removed to provide a space for feeding and approximately positioned hooks are fitted using self-curing acrylic (Figure 7.8). The necessary materials for modifying dentures in this way should always be carried along with other fixation apparatus when called to treat a facial injury away from the main base.

At operation the splints are adapted to the alveolus of each jaw after reduction of the mandibular fracture. Gunning-type splints are frequently employed as an adjunct to some other form of fixation and it may not be possible to fit the lower splint until open reduction and other fixation has been applied. The upper splint is fixed to the alveolus by using an awl to pass a 0.45 mm soft stainless steel wire through the alveolus high up in the canine area on each side and then through an appropriately positioned hole in the palatal portion of the splint. The two free ends on each side are twisted together over the splint, cut short and bent in under one of the hooks or cleats.

The lower splint is attached to the reduced fractured mandible by means of circumferential wires. Care must be taken to avoid passing a circumferential wire close to a fracture site as the wire may be pulled up into the fracture when it is tightened. The most satisfactory method of passing these wires is that described originally by Professor Obwegeser. A suitable curved awl is pushed through the skin beneath the mandible and directed into the mouth on the lingual side of the bone. One end of a length of 0.45 mm soft stainless steel wire is passed through the tip of the awl which is then carefully withdrawn to the lower border of the mandible but not out through the skin. The tip of the awl with the attached wire is guided round the lower border and pushed up into the buccal sulcus where the wire end is detached. The instrument is then withdrawn through the original puncture wound in the skin. The wire is applied close to the bone throughout its passage avoiding the necessity of 'sawing' it through the soft tissues (Figure 7.9a–d).

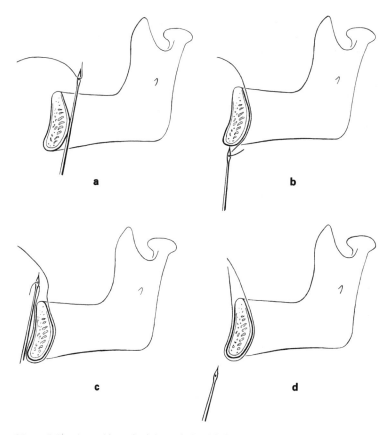

Figure 7.9 a, An awl is pushed through the skin beneath the chin and up into the mouth on the lingual side of the mandible. A length of 0.45 mm soft stainless steel wire is threaded into its tip. **b,** The awl is withdrawn to the lower border of the mandible. **c,** Keeping the awl close to the bone it is passed around the lower border and then pushed up into the buccal sulcus. **d,** The wire is detached from the tip of the awl and the instrument is then withdrawn from the tissues through the external wound

After the splints have been attached to each jaw they are connected by elastic bands or wire loops utilizing the hooks on the buccal surfaces of each splint and intermaxillary fixation is established.

When treatment is completed, the peralveolar and circumferential wires are removed by cutting each wire close to the buccal sulcus and pulling firmly and rapidly. An anaesthetic is not required and if the wire is cut close to the point of mucosal entry this avoids a length of contaminated wire passing through the tissues. In spite of these precautions the passage of the wire during removal occasionally causes infection and it is wise to prescribe antibiotic cover for the procedure.

Gunning-type splints are still widely used as fixation for fractures of the edentulous mandible which justifies describing the technique in some detail. The method is useful for simple fractures treated by surgeons of limited experience. It is, however, a technique which is far from ideal. The splints become exceedingly foul during 4–6 weeks' fixation as a result of food stagnation between the poorly fitting surface of the splint and the mucosa. Apart from the *Candida*-induced stomatitis which results, there is a significant incidence of more serious infection of the wire track within the tissues. These splints are inefficient as a method of immobilization and provide poor control of mobile fractures, particularly when the mandible is very thin. They are unfortunately least efficient in those cases where closed reduction is most desirable.

Selection of the method of fixation

1. In the edentulous mandible reduction and fixation is in the main required for fractures of the angle and body with a view to restoring an adequate denture-bearing area and avoiding facial deformity.
2. Because of the risk of non-union resulting from interference with the periosteal blood supply, reduction should be accomplished with minimal exposure. Many undisplaced fractures require no active treatment.
3. Although Gunning-type splints can be used to achieve fixation after closed reduction, their inherent disadvantages make other methods preferable in all cases requiring active treatment.
4. In otherwise fit patients, open reduction and direct osteosynthesis is the method of choice. Intermaxillary fixation should be avoided wherever possible.
5. The most effective form of osteosynthesis is by non-compression mini-plates. Compression plates offer theoretical advantages which are outweighed by their size in relation to the edentulous bone.
6. When the mandibular body is less than 10 mm in depth, fracture treatment becomes difficult and non-union is more likely. It must be remembered that stable fibrous union may be an acceptable result in the very old or infirm patient. Although

transfixation procedures utilizing Kirschner wires have their protagonists, the method is only occasionally used and the same may be said of systems employing bone clamps and pins. However when there is extensive comminution these methods should be considered.

7. The ultra-thin mandible will not usually unite satisfactorily with conventional methods of reduction and fixation and in these cases autogenous bone grafting as a primary procedure should be the method of choice where the patient's general condition permits.

Chapter 8

Fractures of the condylar region

Fractures involving the mandibular condyle are the only facial bone fractures which involve a synovial joint. Injury to the joint can occur in the absence of any fracture of the articular surfaces. Trauma to this region may therefore be divided into three main types:

1. Contusion: apart from damage to the capsular ligaments such an injury may be accompanied by a synovial effusion, haemarthrosis or tearing of the meniscus. Such injuries are difficult to diagnose without special imaging techniques but they may predispose to later degenerative changes in some cases.
2. Dislocation: irreducible displacement of the condyle from the glenoid fossa is usually anterior or medial. Lateral, posterior or central dislocations rarely occur. A coexisting fracture of the condylar neck is common.
3. Fracture: includes any fracture above the level of the sigmoid notch. Fractures, fracture/dislocations and dislocations of the condyle are all accompanied by varying degrees of contusion. If the fracture extends into the joint space, haemarthrosis and rupture of the meniscus is more likely to occur and such injuries may predispose to later disturbance of function.

It is unfortunate that there are still no clear guidelines for the treatment of fractures of the mandibular condyle. Gerry (1965) observed that 'a patient who has had a condylar fracture cannot be considered to be cured until he is able to masticate easily with the contralateral side of the dentition, which implies the recovery of the condylar excursion'. Clinical experience suggests that many 'successfully' treated cases do not fulfil these criteria.

Conservative management of condylar fractures

Unlike other fractures of the mandible, anatomical reduction and subsequent fixation of condylar fractures is difficult to achieve.

The majority of surgeons have traditionally favoured a conservative approach, avoiding direct disturbance of the fracture site and concentrating on early restoration of function. MacLennan and Simpson (1965), after reviewing several large series of condylar fractures treated in a number of centres, concluded that a good result was achieved by closed conservative management in 93% of cases. A good early functional result does not, however, necessarily mean full recovery of condylar excursion and there is increasing evidence that subsequent joint dysfunction and osteoarthritis can occur (Dahlstrom, Kahnberg and Lindahl, 1989).

A careful prospective study of 76 condylar fractures by Lindahl and Hollender (1977) and Lindahl (1977b) resulted in a number of interesting observations. In the majority of young patients, following fracture of the condyle with displacement, there was a complete anatomical restitution of the temporomandibular articulation within a 2-year period. Amongst teenagers the joint did not return to normality to the same extent and in adults only minor remodelling was observed. Asymmetry of mandibular movement and altered function at the fracture site usually disappeared in children while it persisted or became aggravated in adults. Late symptoms such as clicking and tenderness were rare in children and frequent amongst adults. These authors concluded that

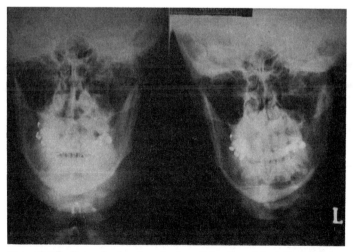

Figure 8.1 Radiographs showing a fracture dislocation of the left condyle in an adult. A functional repair has occurred with obvious residual deformity of the bone contour

remodelling following condylar fractures could be regarded as restitutional in children and adjusting or functional in adults (Figure 8.1).

The important animal experiments of Walker (1960), Boyne (1967) and Choukas *et al.* (1970) were conducted on young monkeys and all demonstrated satisfactory remodelling and healing of experimental condylar fractures, whether surgically reduced or not. It is, however, unwise to extrapolate these results to the adult human as a valid guide to treatment.

Dahlstrom, Kahnberg and Lindahl (1989) have recently completed a 15-year follow-up of a small number of conservatively treated condylar fractures. They have concluded that the older the child the less the capacity for functional remodelling due to reduced resorptive activity. Although adults displayed frequent joint dysfunction, in none was this considered serious. Norman (1982) claimed that many cases of osteoarthritis and recurrent dislocation of the temporomandibular joint were associated with previous trauma while over 60% of cases of ankylosis were the result of previous injury.

Open reduction of condylar fractures

Grossly displaced fracture/dislocations of the condyle, particularly bilateral fractures, are inevitably accompanied by malocclusion in the dentate patient. Simple immobilization by means of intermaxillary fixation does not always achieve a satisfactory reduction of the fracture and malocclusion persists after healing is complete. Functional distraction of the condyle by applying intermaxillary fixation with the bite gagged posteriorly has been recommended in the past but this is not a reliable method. Open surgical reduction and fixation of displaced condylar neck fractures would appear to be a sensible option in such cases. Zide and Kent (1983) have outlined the indications for open reduction as follows:

1. Absolution indications:
   (a) Displacement of condyle into middle cranial fossa.
   (b) Impossibility of restoring occlusion.
   (c) Lateral extracapsular displacement.
   (d) Invasion by foreign body, e.g. missile.
2. Relative indications:
   (a) When intermaxillary fixation is contraindicated for medical reasons.
   (b) Bilateral fracture with associated mid-face fracture.
   (c) Bilateral fracture with severe open bite deformity.

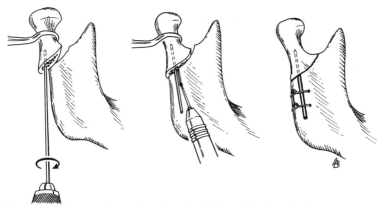

Figure 8.2 Diagram to show a simple method of direct fixation of a displaced condylar neck fracture using a Kirschner wire. (Method devised and reproduced by courtesy of Mr A. E. Brown)

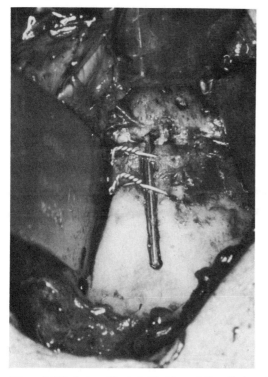

Figure 8.3 Technique illustrated in Figure 8.2 applied to a fracture of the right subcondylar region. (Case treated by Mr A. E. Brown and reproduced by permission of Mr M. D. Awty)

Open reduction is technically difficult and fixation equally so. There is some considerable risk to the branches of the facial nerve although various authors have reported consistent results using transosseous wiring or mini-plates (Tansanen and Lamberg, 1976; Bottcher, Schonberger and Sumnig, 1988; Chuong and Piper, 1988). The method described by Brown and Obeid (1984) is relatively simple and can be used in selected cases (Figures 8.2, 8.3, 8.6 and 8.7).

Major complications

Ankylosis of temporomandibular joint

It has long been recognized that ankylosis of the temporomandibular joint can occur following trauma (El-Mofty, 1972). Equally it is now clear that this is a rare complication occurring in only 0.4% of condylar fractures. The fact that ankylosis appears to be commoner in some parts of the world than in others has led to speculation that there may be a genetic predisposition among some racial groups. Fractures which involve the joint space, particularly in young patients, seem most prone to result in this

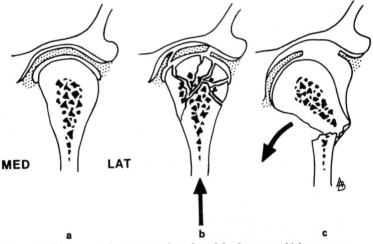

Figure 8.4 Diagrammatic representation of condylar fractures which may cause disruption of the meniscus shown in coronal section. **a**, Normal condyle and meniscus. **b**, Impaction injury giving rise to an intracapsular fracture, haemarthrosis and disruption of the meniscus. **c**, Medial fracture dislocation causing tearing of the meniscus

severe complication although attempts to produce experimental ankylosis in primates have been notably unsuccessful (Markey, Potter and Moffett, 1980; Hohl *et al.*, 1981).

Laskin (1978) has identified predisposing factors as follows:

(a) Age: the major incidence is below the age of 10 years.
(b) Type of injury: intracapsular crushing of the condyle.
(c) Damage to the meniscus: experimental work on large primates has shown that more restriction of movement occurs when an intracapsular fracture is accompanied by excision of the meniscus. Furthermore, remnants of the meniscus can be found in the medial displaced mass of bone, a finding which is common in human cases of bony ankylosis. Disruption of the meniscus is likely to occur in two types of fracture – a severe intracapsular compression injury or a fracture/dislocation (Figure 8.4). Yaillen *et al.* (1979) observed marked degenerative changes in the fossa and condylar head after experimental meniscectomy in Macaca monkeys.

There is no evidence that prolonged immobilization predisposes to either fibrous or bony ankylosis or indeed to restriction of subsequent movement.

Disturbance of growth

A small proportion of children in which the fracture involves the condylar cartilage and the articular surface exhibit subsequent disturbance of growth. In some cases fibrous or bony ankylosis of the temporomandibular joint is an additional complication. This reduces the normal functional movement of the jaw which further inhibits growth. Walker (1957) investigated 50 cases of post-traumatic arrested development of the condyle and found coincident ankylosis in a high proportion. There is an ongoing debate as to whether or not the subcondylar region is a primary growth centre. In practical terms it does not matter whether this part of the mandible is a hormone-dependent primary centre for growth or an area where secondary preferential bone formation takes place as the mandible develops within a functional matrix. The effect of damage to this area of preferential growth is the same – failure of development of the condylar process and a smaller mandible on the affected side.

Treatment of condylar fractures

The methods of treatment of condylar fractures should be based on the clinical and experimental evidence outlined above.

Treatment should be designed to minimize subsequent functional disturbance of the articulation. The difficulties of open reduction and fixation need to be appreciated and where possible a conservative approach preferred.

There are three treatment options:

1. Functional
2. Indirect immobilization
3. Osteosynthesis.

Condylar fractures should be classified according to:

1. Age:
   (a) Under 10 years
   (b) 10–17 years
   (c) Adults.
2. Surgical anatomy:
   (a) Involving joint surface – intracapsular
   (b) Not involving joint surface – extracapsular:
       (i) High condylar neck
       (ii) Low condylar neck.
3. Site:
   (a) Unilateral
   (b) Bilateral.
4. Occlusion:
   (a) Undisturbed
   (b) Malocclusion.

Children under 10 years of age

This group has been shown to be more likely to develop growth disturbance or limitation of movement than other groups. If malocclusion is present entirely as a result of condylar injury, it should be disregarded because spontaneous correction will take place as the dentition develops. Displaced condylar neck fractures will undergo full functional restitution in most cases.

Unilateral and bilateral fractures are treated the same. Treatment should be entirely functional where possible. Indirect immobilization by intermaxillary fixation is indicated for control of pain and should be released after 7–10 days. Where an intracapsular fracture has been diagnosed careful follow-up and monitoring of growth is required and treatment with myofunctional appliances instituted if subsequent mandibular development is reduced.

Adolescents 10–17 years of age

The same principles apply to this group with some modification. If malocclusion is present the capacity for spontaneous correction is less than in the younger group. Malocclusion is therefore an indication for intermaxillary fixation for 2–3 weeks. The dentition at this stage is suitable for the application of simple eyelet wires.

Adults

Unilateral intracapsular fractures

The occlusion is usually undisturbed and the fracture should be treated conservatively without immobilization of the mandible.

Occasionally slight malocclusion is noted, particularly when there is an associated effusion in the joint, in which case simple intermaxillary fixation with eyelet wires should be applied for 2–3 weeks.

Unilateral condylar neck fractures

If the fracture is undisplaced the occlusion will generally be undisturbed and no active treatment is necessary. A fracture/dislocation will often induce significant malocclusion due to shortening of the ramus height and premature contact of the molar teeth on that side. A low condylar neck fracture is probably best treated by open reduction in these circumstances.

In the case of a high condylar neck fracture with extensive displacement and malocclusion, intermaxillary fixation is applied and maintained until stable bony union has occurred, i.e. 3–4 weeks. In spite of maintaining the occlusion by intermaxillary fixation relapse may take place when the fixation is removed. As this is usually slight it can be corrected by a combination of occlusal grinding and spontaneous adaptation.

Bilateral intracapsular fractures

The occlusion is usually slightly deranged in these cases. The degree of displacement of the two condyles may not be the same and it is best to immobilize the mandible for the 3–4 weeks required for stable union. It used to be thought that this would predispose to chronic limitation of movement but post reduction physiotherapy in the form of simple jaw exercises is effective in preventing this.

Bilateral condylar neck fractures

These fractures present the major problem in treatment. There is usually considerable displacement of one side or the other. Even if displacement is not evident when first seen, the fractures are inherently unstable and functional treatment is contraindicated. Although the application of intermaxillary fixation will establish the occlusion, it will not reliably reduce the fracture on both sides. Operative reduction of at least one of the fractures to restore the ramus height is desirable (Figures 8.5–8.9). In the case of bilateral high condylar neck fractures where operative reduction is likely to be difficult, intermaxillary fixation should be applied for up to 6 weeks. If strong arch bars or even cap splints are applied this will allow the use of intermittent intermaxillary elastics at night for several weeks after fixation is removed. This technique may encourage better functional remodelling.

Although ankylosis of the temporomandibular joint itself does not occur with condylar neck fractures, exuberant callus formation

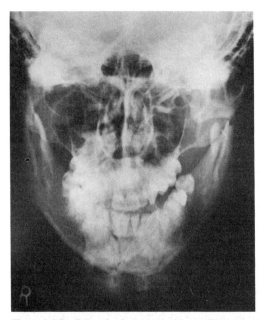

Figure 8.5 Radiograph of a patient with mandibular fractures resulting from direct violence to the symphysis. Fractures have occurred at the symphysis and both subcondylar regions. There is considerable medial displacement of the left condyle and shortening of the ramus. The 'gagged' occlusion is clearly demonstrated

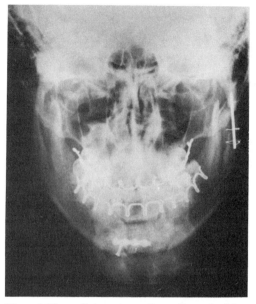

Figure 8.6 Immediate postoperative radiograph of the patient shown in Figure 8.5. A lag screw and a mini-plate have been used to immobilize the reduced symphyseal fracture. The left condyle has been repositioned and fixed internally by the method shown in Figures 8.2 and 8.3

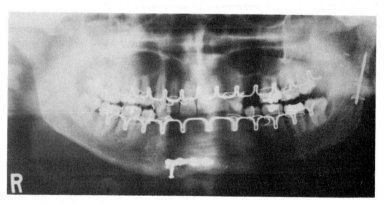

Figure 8.7 The immediate postoperative panoral tomogram of the patient in Figures 8.5 and 8.6

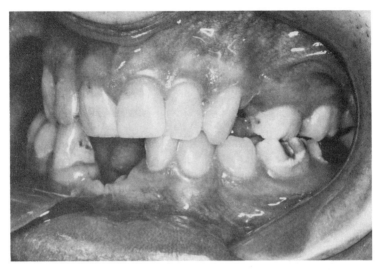

Figure 8.8 Intra-oral postoperative photograph of the patient in Figures 8.5–8.7 showing good restoration of the occlusion

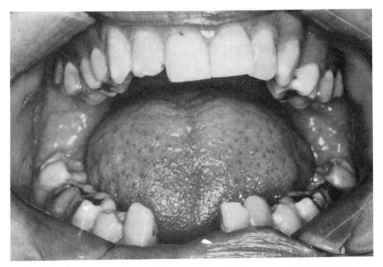

Figure 8.9 Intra-oral photograph showing the opening achieved within 2 weeks of fixation in the patient shown in Figures 8.5–8.8. No mandibular deviation is apparent

round grossly displaced fragments may cause extra-articular interference with joint excursion.

When a bilateral fracture of this nature is associated with a major mid-facial fracture, operative reduction of both sides is desirable. It should be appreciated that this represents a considerable amount of operating time even in skilled hands. The situation may be temporarily saved by the use of extra-oral fixation utilizing a box-frame or halo.

Chapter 9

Fractures of the mandible in children

Fractures of the mandible are uncommon in children owing to the fact that the bone is resilient at this age and considerable force is required to effect a fracture. The line of demarcation between the medulla and cortex is less well defined than in adults whereas the ratio of bone to tooth substance is high (Khosla and Boren, 1971). Incomplete dysjunction in the form of a 'greenstick' fracture is therefore more likely and there is a greater risk of damage to developing teeth than in later years (Figure 9.1). Ranta and Ylipaavalniemi (1973) carried out a long-term investigation of teeth involved in mandibular fractures occurring before the age of

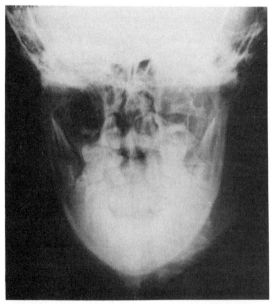

Figure 9.1 A 'greenstick' fracture of the right condyle noted in a postero-anterior radiograph

12 years, and observed disturbed formation in 72% of teeth directly involved in the line of fracture. They also noted from other surveys that between 25 and 48% of teeth involved in the fracture line in adults exhibited pulp necrosis.

Keniry (1971) in a survey of the literature found that between 8.3% and 15% of jaw fractures occurred in children under the age of 15 years. According to MacLennan (1956) only 1% of mandibular fractures happened before the age of 6 years.

The treatment of mandibular fractures in children before puberty is generally of a conservative nature because of the rapidity of healing and the adaptive potential of the bone and its contained dentition.

There are a few special factors which need to be taken into account in managing these injuries.

Interference with growth potential

The normal growth of the mandible will be disturbed if unerupted permanent teeth or teeth germs are lost, because the alveolus will not develop normally in the areas affected. Damage to the growth potential will be more severe in the event of infection of the fracture site.

McGuirt and Salisbury (1987) carried out a careful cephalo-metric analysis of 28 children who had experienced mandibular fractures at sites other than the condyle and found the mandibular unit length to be less than expected in 67%. One-third of the patients with fractures in the tooth-bearing portion of the mandible had specific dental complications.

The capacity for preferential growth in the sub-condylar region may be seriously compromised by high condylar fractures, particularly if function is restricted as a result of fibrous or bony ankylosis of the temporomandibular joint. The treatment of these injuries has been discussed in Chapter 8.

Fixation in the deciduous and mixed dentition period

If the severity and displacement of the fracture are of sufficient degree to warrant immobilization of the mandible, some modification of technique is required because of the presence of unerupted or partially erupted teeth of the permanent dentition and deciduous teeth of variable mobility.

Fixation independent of the teeth

1. In the very young with unerupted or very few deciduous teeth MacLennan (1956) recommends the use of an overall Gunning-type splint for the lower jaw alone. This is constructed as a trough lined with black gutta percha and retained by two circumferential wires.
2. Where some occlusion is present but there is widespread caries or loose deciduous teeth the mandible may be suspended by circumferential wires on each side linked to circumzygomatic wires from above.
3. A simple elasticated bandage chin support may be used in cases with minimal displacement where jaw movement is nevertheless painful.

Fixation utilizing the teeth

1. Cap splints can be constructed for the mixed dentition but retention tends to be inadequate, particularly if partially erupted teeth are present. It is necessary to reinforce the cement bond with circumferential wires tied over the splint on each side.
2. Where there are sufficient firm erupted deciduous and permanent teeth, eyelet wires or arch bars can be used. It is

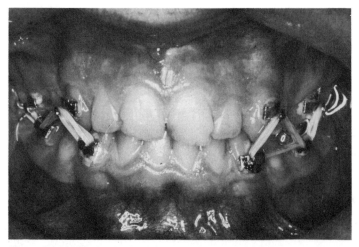

Figure 9.2 Modified orthodontic brackets fixed to the teeth of a young patient by acid-etching and composite bonding. Intermaxillary elastics have been used to immobilize the mandible which had a relatively undisplaced fracture of the left angle

often difficult to fix wires firmly to deciduous molars and canines but this task is made easier by using thinner more flexible soft stainless steel wires of 0.35 mm diameter. Similarly, a light arch bar of German silver without hooks is more easily adapted to the irregular dentition and this should be attached to the teeth by similar 0.35 mm diameter wire ligatures. Orthodontic brackets bonded directly to the teeth may be used in simple fractures (Figure 9.2).

Unerupted teeth

In patients below the age of 9 or 10 years the body of the mandible is congested with developing teeth. It is unsafe to apply transosseous wires or to insert bone pins or plates in these circumstances. In exceptional instances such as gross displacement of a symphysis or angle fracture the lower border may be wired with caution – bone plates and pins are contraindicated.

Healing and remodelling

Mandibular fractures in children heal very rapidly and some fractures are stable within a week, and firmly united within 3 weeks. If at the time the fracture is first seen the fragments are firm, but not perfectly reduced, it is as well to accept some slight imperfection in the reduction rather than refracture the mandible with possible damage to developing teeth. Similarly, some imperfection in reduction can be accepted when a fresh fracture is treated, as in each of the above circumstances continuing growth and eruption of teeth will compensate in most cases for the imperfect alignment of the fragments.

Finally, it should be emphasized that a prolonged follow-up period is required following most fractures of the mandible in children in order to be sure that there are no long-term effects on both mandibular growth and the normal development of the permanent dentition. There are often damaged teeth associated with fractures in this age group and close cooperation with the paedodontist, orthodontist and the patient's general dental practitioner is of vital importance.

Chapter 10

Postoperative care

Operative treatment of injuries to structures associated with the patient's airway gives rise to special postoperative problems. Those problems are compounded if the jaws have to be immobilized before the patient has fully regained conscious control of the airway. The recent trend towards treatment of mandibular fractures by direct osteosynthesis has made postoperative care simpler and safer in the main.

Postoperative care may be divided into three phases:

1. The immediate postoperative phase when the patient is recovering from the general anaesthetic.
2. The intermediate phase before clinical bony union has become established.
3. The late postoperative phase which includes removal of fixation, bite rehabilitation, physiotherapy and long-term observation of the dentition in particular.

Immediate postoperative phase

Most maxillofacial units have a special high dependency or intensive care unit to which patients are transferred from the operating theatre and there they are kept under skilled nursing supervision until they are fully recovered from the anaesthetic and fit to be transferred back to their ward. In the absence of such facilities an experienced nurse should remain with the patient until recovery is complete.

If intermaxillary fixation has been carried out it is prudent to have available at the patient's bedside instruments such as scissors, wire cutters, screwdrivers, etc. so that the fixation can be removed in an emergency. It is also essential that good lighting is provided and that accessory lighting is available in case of a power failure. Patients should be returned from the theatre with a nasopharyngeal airway in position and this should be left *in situ* until the patient recovers consciousness. Control of the tongue in the unconscious patient can be effected if the surgeon inserts a tongue suture at the end of operation. Physical control of the tongue in an unconscious patient is only required if there has been extensive soft-tissue injury to the oropharynx or in a patient who is expected to remain cerebrally irritated after recovery. Many patients in this category will have had elective tracheostomy or prolonged endotracheal intubation. A tongue suture passed transversely across the dorsum of the tongue may be employed as an additional safeguard.

Patients should be nursed lying on their sides during recovery to enable any saliva or oozing blood to escape from the mouth. An efficient suction apparatus must be at the patient's bedside and to the sucker nozzle a length of ⅛ inch (3 mm) rubber or polythene tubing is attached. This enables the nurse to pass the tube down the nasopharyngeal airway or the nares to suck out the nasopharynx. The rubber or polythene suction tube can also be passed along the buccal sulcus to keep this area free of secretions.

Postoperative vomiting should not occur if it has been possible for the patient to be correctly prepared for operation. If a genuine emergency operation is required, there may be significant amounts of recently swallowed blood as well as food within the stomach. In these circumstances it will be necessary to evacuate the stomach contents before anaesthetizing the patient. Skilled anaesthesia will reduce the incidence of postoperative vomiting to negligible proportions. If vomiting should occur in the presence of intermaxillary fixation, it presents no danger to the airway if adequate nursing care is present. It is, however, extremely unpleasant for the patient but much less so if intermaxillary fixation has been avoided.

Patients with external pin fixation need careful nursing while restless during recovery to avoid damage to the apparatus.

Intermediate postoperative care

General supervision

Patients who have sustained a maxillofacial injury and who are in hospital will not normally require high dependency care after the first 24 hours. They should be carefully examined at both a morning and evening ward round. The occlusion should be checked as early as possible. Direct osteosynthesis carries with it a greater risk of malalignment. Unacceptable reduction needs to be corrected at an early stage, by further surgery if necessary.

Intermaxillary fixation must be inspected to ensure the postoperative reduction has been maintained and fixation has not become loose. The clinical observations must be supported by early postoperative radiographs to confirm that satisfactory reduction and fixation has been achieved.

An adequately reduced and immobilized mandibular fracture is relatively painless and the postoperative oedema rapidly subsides. Any increase in swelling, particularly if accompanied by signs of active infection, requires immediate attention.

Posture

Patients with a fracture of the mandible find it more comfortable if they are in the sitting position with the chin well forward and providing there is no contraindication to this posture such as a fractured vertebra the conscious patient should be nursed in this position. The comatose or stuporose patient is best nursed lying on the side so that saliva and blood can dribble out of the mouth.

Sedation

If the fracture has been adequately reduced and effectively immobilized, the patient will experience very little pain and postoperative analgesics are seldom indicated and should not be administered routinely.

Morphine and its derivatives are contraindicated in patients with maxillofacial injuries. These drugs depress the respiratory centre and cough reflex and for these reasons alone they are potentially dangerous if given to patients whose jaws are immobilized. The use of any powerful analgesic may mask a deteriorating level of consciousness and morphine derivatives cause constriction of the pupil which obscures the pupillary changes indicative of a rise in intracranial pressure. Patients with mandibular fractures frequently have other injuries apart from associated head injury and it is important that the physical signs of, for example intra-abdominal bleeding, are not suppressed by analgesics before the patient's condition has been fully evaluated. Patients who are cerebrally irritated require sedation which is best achieved by intravenous diazepam. This drug sedates the patient well and has very few disadvantageous other effects. The dose is adjusted according to the patient's response to 5 mg increments. It should be remembered that restlessness in a semi-conscious patient may be due to airway difficulties or a distended bladder.

Prevention of infection

Fractures of the tooth-bearing portion of the mandible are liable to infection and prophylactic antibiotics should be given. Unless contraindicated penicillin is the drug of choice and many surgeons now add metronidazole to the regime. If healing is proceeding well, antibiotics can be discontinued 5 days after immobilization of the fracture. Simple closed fractures of the condylar neck do not require prophylactic antibiotics.

Oral hygiene

Effective oral hygiene also plays an important part in the prevention of infection of the fracture line. The conscious patient is given hot normal saline mouthwashes following every meal and patients whose fractures are immobilized by any of the wiring techniques (direct, eyelet, or arch) or by silver-copper alloy cap splints can keep the fixation clean by using a toothbrush in the usual manner.

Nash and Addy (1980) have shown that a 0.2% chlorhexidine gluconate mouthwash significantly reduces bacterial counts and improves plaque control in patients with intermaxillary fixation.

If the patient is too ill to cooperate in these simple measures to promote oral hygiene, the mouth must be cleaned by the nursing staff after every meal using normal saline solution which is squirted into the mouth with a Higginson syringe. Care must be taken not to direct the stream of fluid down the site of any compounded fractures, so introducing infection. Cap splints can be cleaned with a 1–4% sodium bicarbonate solution on cotton-wool swabs held in forceps. Rubber bands may become soiled with food and should be changed when this occurs.

In spite of the theoretical advantages of intermaxillary elastics when cap splints are used, there is no doubt that wire loops are more hygienic and for this reason many operators prefer them. The lips should at all times be kept lubricated with petroleum jelly to prevent them becoming dry and sticking together. If the lips are in any way excoriated and sore as they may be after operative reduction and fixation, 1% hydrocortisone ointment can be applied with benefit.

Immediately following operation the saliva tends to become thick and difficult to control. This condition may persists for the first few days after injury. It is much more difficult for a patient to cope with this if intermaxillary fixation has had to be used. The thickened saliva and congealed blood tend to block the interstices between the teeth and hinder oral respiration. The lips tend to stick together which adds to the problem. It is during this period that good nursing can do much to aid rapid recovery. The lips and mouth should be cleaned with moist saline swabs at regular intervals and the lips regularly lubricated with steroid-containing ointment or petroleum jelly.

Feeding

The problem of providing a patient suffering from a maxillofacial injury with adequate nutrition varies according to whether the subject is conscious and cooperative or is uncooperative due to a low level of consciousness or to cerebral irritation.

The conscious cooperative patient

The majority of patients with a fractured mandible can be fed by mouth even though their jaws are immobilized. Depending upon the size of the gaps in their fixation they can eat a semi-solid or a liquid diet.

A diet of 2000–2500 calories is adequate for most patients' nutritional requirements. A liquid or semi-solid diet is uninteresting and tedious to consume and for this reason patients should be encouraged to eat a little and often. The balance of the diet should be decided in consultation with a dietitian who will generally encourage patients to eat as much of their normal food as can be prepared by an electric food mixer or liquidizer. Milk and milk products are encouraged for regular daily consumption. The diet usually needs to be supplemented with vitamins, iron preparations and high-calorie protein preparations such as Complan. Every effort should be made to maintain the patient's interest in the diet by the use of flavouring agents and the food should be presented in as attractive a manner as possible.

A feeding cup with a spout to which a suitable length of soft plastic tubing is attached enables a patient to feed himself by passing the end of the tubing through a gap in the fixation or round the back of the lower teeth. Flexible drinking straws are also very helpful to enable a patient to drink from a vessel.

The unconscious or uncooperative patient

Fluid balance

A fluid balance chart should be kept for all patients suffering from maxillofacial injuries until such time as the clinician in charge of the case is satisfied that an adequate fluid intake is being voluntarily ingested by the patient. The normal daily intake of water is about 3000 ml and the output is made up of 1500 ml of insensible loss by evaporation from the skin, sweating, etc. and 1500 ml of urine.

It should be remembered that all forms of trauma and operations provoke a complex metabolic disturbance which varies directly with the magnitude and duration of the trauma or operation. This consists essentially of an inability to excrete water and salt with an increased metabolism and excretion of potassium and nitrogen. The impairment of water excretion lasts 24–36 hours and is characterized by low output of urine of high specific gravity. The impairment of secretion of sodium lasts 4–6 days and after 24 hours there is marked lowering of sodium and chlorine in the urine. There is an increased excretion of potassium which lasts 24–48 hours due to mobilization and excretion of intracellular potassium. The increased nitrogen excretion is due to the breakdown of tissue. These changes are a normal response to trauma and in most cases the disturbances are slight and do not require any action. Most patients with a fractured mandible are on a normal diet and fluid intake up to the time of injury and are therefore in normal electrolyte balance. Usually such patients can return to an adequate fluid intake by mouth as soon as the fracture is immobilized and such cases present no fluid balance problems. In conscious patients the fluid intake can be left to the desires of the patient, for normally the kidneys have enormous flexibility of function and can excrete excess salt or fluid from the body. This flexibility, as already stated, is temporarily lost following trauma and operation. Intravenous fluids lack the safeguard of the patient's desire for fluid and therefore the amount administered has to be accurately assessed by the surgeon.

In a patient unable to swallow due to a severe mandibular fracture, considerable dehydration can occur in 24–48 hours especially in elderly patients. If the patient is capable of taking fluid by mouth, it is unnecessary to employ any other route, but if for some reason the patient cannot swallow, enteral or parenteral fluid therapy must be instituted.

Enteral fluid therapy
Enteral fluid therapy is effected by passing fluid into the stomach via a transnasal gastric tube. Considerable advances have been made in recent years in this form of feeding mainly derived from experience with burn injuries. All the patient's nutritional requirements may now be administered via a soft very thin flexible

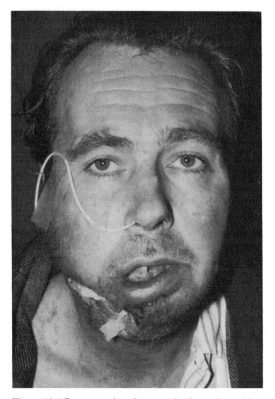

Figure 10.1 Postoperative photograph of a patient with a severe gunshot wound involving the right mandible. An ultra-thin flexible nasogastric tube has been passed to permit enteral feeding with minimal discomfort for the patient

nasogastric tube using specially constituted food preparations injected slowly under pressure (Silk, 1980; Brown, 1981) (Figure 10.1). If a nasogastric tube is passed in order to feed the patient it is essential to take a chest radiograph to ensure that it is in the stomach before any food is given. Occasionally these tubes are inadvertently passed into the trachea.

Parenteral fluid therapy
Parenteral fluid therapy is administered by an intravenous drip and the greatest risk with this form of therapy is that of overloading the patient with water while the normal kidney flexibility of function is temporarily impaired as a result of the trauma and/or operation. It is exceptional for patients who have

sustained a fractured mandible to require intravenous fluid in the postoperative period in the absence of some complication such as protracted unconsciousness, though intravenous blood or other fluid may have to be given immediately following the accident if the patient is shocked. As already stated, shock is rare following fracture of the mandible and if present is usually due to some asociated injury. In all instances patients should revert to oral fluid and feeding as soon as possible.

Late postoperative care

Testing of union and removal of fixation

Fractures of the body and ramus of the mandible treated by rigid osteosynthesis will not normally have had intermaxillary fixation applied for other than a short period designed to minimize postoperative discomfort. Although these methods produce a strong clinically stable union more rapidly than non-rigid fixation, some care is needed in the management of the early stages. Patients should be kept on a soft diet for the first 2 weeks and carefully monitored in order that wound infection, should it occur, is recognized at an early stage. In some treatment centres plates are routinely removed after 6 months whereas in others they are left as permanent implants unless they become exposed or infected. There is evidence to suggest that routine removal of internal fixation is unnecessary. Larger plates, e.g. those designed for compression osteosynthesis, are more likely to become exposed. Similarly the larger interface with vital tissue is more likely, in the longer term, to become infected from blood-borne organisms. All plates and certainly all transosseous wires are probably better regarded as permanent implants unless they cause trouble. Removal is indicated because of infection, exposure to the mouth, close and prominent proximity to the skin or interference with the subsequent design of a prosthesis.

When intermaxillary fixation has been employed, it is left until sufficient time has elapsed for stable clinical union to be expected. It is then dismantled in part to allow the fracture site to be tested by gentle manipulation. If the fracture is stable in normal function, intermaxillary fixation is discontinued and the fracture examined again 1 week later. Some movement across the fracture is acceptable when intermaxillary wires are removed. The amount of acceptable mobility is a matter of clinical experience which is not difficult to acquire.

All current methods used to apply intermaxillary fixation allow the wires to be removed without disturbing the fixation to the teeth. This gives the clinician the option to immobilize the mandible for a further period with minimal inconvenience to the patient. The exception to this arises when Gunning-type splints are used for edentulous fractures. It is then necessary to remove the whole splint before the fracture can be tested – an additional disadvantage of the technique.

When the fracture is satisfactorily united the fixation apparatus is removed in its entirety. Wire ligatures and eyelets should be unwound a few turns to loosen them and the wire cut in such a way that there are no residual obstructions to smooth withdrawal. Nevertheless the process is uncomfortable for the patient. Local anaesthesia over a wide area is impractical but inhalation relative analgesia can be employed with advantage.

Peralveolar and circumferential wires are removed by cutting one end close to the gum and pulling on the opposite end of the wire. No anaesthetic is necessary, but it is essential to cut the wire cleanly, for a jagged end of wire causes pain as it is pulled through the tissues. The mouth should be cleaned with antiseptic such as 1% chlorhexidine gluconate solution before pulling out the wire to avoid introducing infection deep into the tissues. It is helpful as an additional safeguard against infection to administer an antibiotic such as 1 mega unit of penicillin at this time.

Cap splints are removed with an old pair of upper Reid forceps. One blade is placed on the edge of the splint near the gingival margin and the other blade on the occlusal surface of the splint. The handles of the forceps are approximated to squeeze the two blades together and the underlying copper cement is cracked. This manoeuvre is carried out all round the splint and when it is loose it is lifted off the teeth. The residual black copper cement should be removed as soon as possible as it tends to get excessively hard when bathed in saliva for any length of time. Special care should be taken to remove copper cement from the occlusal surfaces of the teeth, for its presence may derange the bite and cause the patient to adopt a bite of convenience. This tends to throw strain on the newly healed fracture. Extra-oral pins are removed by gripping each pin with heavy pliers and removing it with a rotatory, pulling movement. The skin surrounding the pins should be well cleaned with an antiseptic before removing them to avoid infection.

Adjustment of occlusion

Little adjustment of the occlusion is required when direct or eyelet wiring has been employed as the cusps are placed in their correct position under direct vision at the time of immobilization of the fracture.

Some slight adjustment to the occlusion is required, however, when cap splints have been employed, for no matter how accurately they have been constructed there is, of necessity, a layer of splint metal and a layer of cement over the cusp of each tooth incorporated in the splint. Slight derangement of the occlusion can often be overcome by allowing the patient to masticate normally, for usually there is sufficient elasticity in the recently healed fracture to allow the occlusion to correct itself.

More gross abnormalities of the occlusion are treated by selective grinding of the cusps. Special problems arise when only a small number of teeth are present in either jaw, for the patient tends to assume a bite of convenience. Such cases should be fitted with partial upper and lower dentures as soon as possible to stabilize the bite. Patients with fractures of the edentulous mandible can seldom wear their original lower dentures and new ones are required when the fracture is healed.

Mobilization of the temporomandibular joint

Patients seldom have any difficulty in moving their temporomandibular joints following a protracted period of immobilization of the mandible, and usually no special treatment is required on removing the fixation beyond encouraging movement. The function of the temporomandibular joint may, however, be adversely affected in certain fractures of the condyle particularly when intracapsular. Post-traumatic disorders of the temporomandibular joint are probably much more common than has hitherto been recognized (Norman, 1982) and indeed the overall mobility and closing force of the mandible may be significantly reduced by fractures other than those involving the condyle (Wood, 1980).

Anaesthesia and paraesthesia of the lower lip

If the inferior dental nerve is involved in the fracture the damage may take the form of a neuropraxia or neurotmesis and the period for recovery of sensation will, of course, depend on the nature and degree of the damage to the nerve. A neuropraxia usually recovers in about 6 weeks, but a neurotmesis may take 18 months. Following severe damage to the nerve complete recovery may not occur and the patient will complain of a slightly altered sensation on the affected side. However, some degree of sensation in the lip always occurs, as the area of the lower lip supplied by the inferior dental nerve has an accessory sensory supply from the mylohyoid nerve. The lingual nerve is seldom damaged in civilian-type mandibular fractures but if the nerve is severed sensation in the anterior two-thirds of the tongue is seldom re-established. Microneural repair of both the inferior dental nerve and lingual nerve can now be carried out in specialized centres. The results are sufficiently encouraging to justify the procedure in selected cases.

Teeth and supporting tissues

Fixation methods which involve attachments to the teeth need to distribute the load so as to avoid excessive traction on individual segments of the dentition. Otherwise significant damage to the periodontal ligament will occur which may be irreversible. After removal of eyelet wires, arch bars or cap splints, vigorous attention to oral hygiene is essential and the patient should be instructed accordingly. Where teeth have been retained in the line of fracture, localized periodontal breakdown may need specific periodontal treatment to obviate further deterioration. Fortunately the periodontal ligament undergoes rapid repair after trauma and is reconstituted within a period of 2 weeks in the majority of cases (Andreason and Andreason, 1990).

Teeth, whether directly or indirectly involved in the fracture, may have been devitalised. Indeed studies have shown that up to 50% of involved teeth undergo pulp necrosis (Ranta and Ylipaavalniemi, 1973). Such teeth are often in a denervated section of the mandible and standard vitality tests are unreliable. Careful postoperative monitoring of the dentition is most important and unfortunately often neglected.

When teeth have been lost, replacement by fixed or removable prostheses should be part of the overall treatment plan. In many countries restorative dentistry is a Cinderella specialty in maxillofacial treatment centres. In view of the frequency of mandibular and other facial fractures and the considerable damage to the dentition which accrues, it is surprising that health authorities do not more widely recognize that restoration and rehabilitation of the dentition is an integral part of the management of the maxillofacial injury.

Chapter 11

Complications

Serious complications arising as a result of a fracture of the mandible are rare providing the fracture has been competently treated. Minor complications are, however, more common than is generally accepted (Afzelius and Rosen, 1980). Complications may be considered under two headings:

1. Complications arising during primary treatment.
2. Late complications.

Complications arising during primary treatment

Misapplied fixation

The increased use of bone plates, particularly in the tooth-bearing portion of the mandible, has increased the complication rate during primary treatment. Compression plates demand screws of sufficient length to impinge on the inner cortex. Care is needed to avoid the inferior dental canal and to avoid damage to the roots of teeth. The risk of damage to structures within the body of the mandible is less when the screw engages only the outer cortex as is the case with non-compression mini-plates.

Rigid osteosynthesis can distort the anatomical alignment of the mandible leading to significant alteration of the occlusion. Should this occur a decision must be made as to whether the malalignment can be corrected by later occlusal adjustment or whether a second corrective operation should be performed.

Osteosynthesis by transosseous wires is technically easier and damage to internal structures should be avoidable. Nevertheless ill-judged direction of drill holes can cause problems. Circumferential wires, particularly those used to retain Gunning-type splints, must be carefully located. If the circumferential wire is close to a fracture line it may inadvertently be drawn up into the fracture giving rise to displacement of the bone fragments, damage to the inferior dental bundle and inadequate retention of the splint.

The correct insertion of pins for external fixation is even more hazardous in unskilled hands. The pins have to be inserted without the advantage of direct exposure of the bone. They may impinge on nerves, blood vessels or teeth. They may split the bone fragment if inserted too near the lower border and they may fail to penetrate sufficient bone substance to remain secure during the required period of fixation.

Infection

Infection of the fracture site resulting in necrosis or osteomyelitis of the mandible is rare (Figure 11.1). When teeth are retained in the fracture line there is always some risk of infection and for this

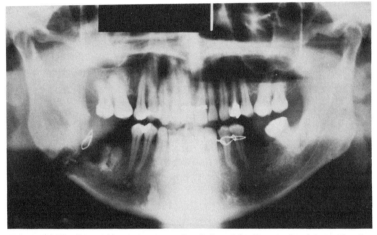

Figure 11.1 Radiographic appearance of an infected fracture at the right angle of the mandible. An upper border wire had been previously inserted. At least two sequestra are delineated within the radiolucency caused by the infection

reason prophylactic antibiotics should be prescribed. Lowering of the patient's local or general resistance will predispose to infection. Pathological fracture such as may be caused by the presence of a benign or malignant neoplasm is a good example of diminished local resistance to bacterial invasion. Debilitated patients, diabetics and patients on steroid therapy are more likely to develop infected fracture sites because of lowered general resistance.

Some of the most severe infections of fracture sites are seen as a result of injudicious surgical interference, such as transosseous wiring of a fracture already infected.

Nerve damage

Anaesthesia of the lower lip as a result of neuropraxia or neurotmesis of the inferior dental nerve is the most common complication of fracture of the body of the mandible. The recovery of sensation in the lower lip depends on the nature of the original damage to the nerve. While anaesthesia is present the patient should be warned of the danger of burning the lower lip with hot drinks or cigarettes.

Facial nerve damage may complicate some fractures of the ramus and condyle, either as a result of a penetrating injury severing branches of the nerve, or blunt trauma causing a neuropraxia. In the latter event recovery of the resultant nerve weakness usually takes place fairly rapidly. If the facial nerve is severed modern microsurgical techniques are often successful in restoring function but it is most important to perform the repair at the same time as the facial laceration is explored and sutured. It is much more difficult to restore continuity and function as a later secondary procedure.

Displaced teeth and foreign bodies

Teeth or portions of dentures are occasionally inhaled and, when missing, must be accounted for. If this is not possible the chest must be radiographed and if a foreign body is present it should be recovered by bronchoscopy.

Fragments of teeth or glass are not infrequently buried in the soft tissues of the lip. They may be difficult to locate in swollen tissues but may become infected if left. If an abscess does occur, the site of pus formation locates the foreign body which is then usually removed easily when the abscess is opened and drained.

Pulpitis

Damaged teeth may develop pulpitis or apical infection during the period of fixation. Such teeth are relatively easy to treat if arch bars or eyelet wires have been employed. If a tooth becomes painful under a cap splint it is occasionally necessary to remove the root portion via a buccal transalveolar surgical approach. The tooth is sectioned at the cervical margin and the crown left within the cap splint.

Gingival and periodontal complications

Some degree of local gingivitis is inevitable when the fixation employed involves interdental wires or cap splints. The gingival reaction may be very severe when acrylic resin is used to attach cap splints to the teeth. Gingivitis is usually not a serious problem and responds to local measures.

A more serious periodontal problem can result from applying too much interdental force to individual teeth from eyelet wires or arch bars. The lower incisors are most vulnerable and may be partially extruded or even lost. The complication can be avoided by spreading the load more widely and evenly by additional eyelets or arch bar ligatures, and by avoiding the application of wires to suspect teeth.

Drug reactions

Allergic reactions occur from time to time usually to antibiotics. These are fortunately in the main fairly mild but the clinician must recognize the complication at an early stage, discontinue all drugs which might be incriminated and prescribe an antihistamine such as oral chlorpheniramine maleate (Piriton) 4 mg t.d.s.

Later complications

Malunion

Post reduction radiographs must always be taken and should these reveal an unacceptable malposition of the fragments, this should be corrected as soon as possible by a further operation if necessary.

When fixation is removed there should be no derangement of the occlusion. Unfortunately from time to time some disturbance is found to be present. Such minor malunion is more common after cap splints have been employed and results either from failure to seat the splints evenly when originally cemented into place, or from faulty laboratory technique producing variation in the thickness of the metal casting. If fixation is removed at the stage of clinical union when the callus is still soft, minor discrepancies in the occlusion will often correct themselves as the patient starts to use the jaws again. The process of readjustment may be helped by selective occlusal grinding.

Occasionally cases may be seen where inadequate reduction has resulted in gross derangement of the occlusion and deformity of the face. This situation may also arise when a patient has had no treatment at all for the fractured mandible, either because he did not seek treatment at the time of injury, or because other more serious injuries prevented treatment or diagnosis. The mandible has an impressive capacity to heal itself and providing some bone contact is present, malunion is more likely than non-union. Gross occlusal derangement and facial deformity requires operative reconstruction usually in the form of refracture. Occasionally a formal planned osteotomy or ostectomy may be required. When the jaw is refractured to correct malunion it is wise to pack autogenous cancellous bone chips obtained from the iliac crest around the newly approximated bone ends. If this is not done the diminished blood supply at the site of the original injury may predispose to further delayed union. Occasionally alloplastic onlays may be indicated particularly when there is asymmetry.

Delayed and non-union

Delayed union

If the time taken for a mandibular fracture to unite is unduly protracted it is referred to as a case of 'delayed union'. The term is difficult to define precisely as fractures heal at different rates, but if union is delayed beyond the expected time for that particular fracture (taking the site and the patient's age into consideration) it must be assumed that the healing process has been disturbed. This may be the result of local factors such as infection, or general factors such as osteoporosis or nutritional deficiency. Providing the fracture site becomes stable so that jaw function can be resumed, no active intervention is necessary in the short term. A fracture in which fibrous union has occurred will frequently progress to slow bony consolidation during the ensuing 12 months after injury. Fibrous union may be an acceptable result in an elderly edentulous patient. However, in a younger dentate individual, prosthetic replacement of missing teeth is impractical if any mobility at a fracture site remains and at some point non-union has to be accepted and treated.

Non-union

Non-union means that the fracture is not only not united but will not unite on its own. Radiographs show rounding off and sclerosis of the bone ends, a condition referred to as eburnation. Non-union includes the condition of fibrous union referred to previously when there is a degree of stability.

Non-union may occur in a number of circumstances some of which are preventable. The theoretically preventable causes of non-union are as follows:

1. Infection of the fracture site.
2. Inadequate immobilization.
3. Unsatisfactory apposition of bone ends with interposition of soft tissue.

The remaining causes of non-union may be impossible or very difficult to overcome and are as follows:

1. The ultra-thin edentulous mandible in an elderly debilitated patient.
2. Loss of bone and soft tissue as a result of severe trauma, e.g. missile injury.
3. Inadequate blood supply to fracture site, e.g. after radiotherapy.
4. The presence of bone pathology, e.g. a malignant neoplasm.
5. General disease, e.g. osteoporosis, severe nutritional deficiency, disorders of calcium metabolism.

Treatment
A moderate delay in union is treated by prolonging the period of immobilization. Once non-union is accepted and if the bone ends are still approximated, the fracture line should be explored surgically and any obvious impediment to healing such as a sequestrum or devitalized tooth removed. The bone ends are then freshened, the wound closed and the jaw is immobilized once again. If there is any doubt concerning the health of the bone ends autogenous cancellous bone chips should be obtained from the iliac crest and packed around the fracture site.

If radiographs of a non-union show marked eburnation of the bone ends or excessive bone loss, a formal bone graft of cortico-cancellous bone will be required. It is important to eliminate active infection from the site before employing a bone graft although if the obvious cause of the infection has been eliminated, a bone graft inserted at the same operation will usually be successful. In these circumstances metronidazole 500 mg every 8 hours given intravenously in an infusion is a most useful prophylactic antibiotic.

Derangement of the temporomandibular joint

Conservative treatment of the fractured mandibular condyle frequently leaves a state of malunion at the fracture site.

Post-traumatic temporomandibular joint problems are not uncommon (see Chapter 8).

Late problems with transosseous wires and plates

Transosseous wires at the upper border may cause symptoms, particularly if covered by a denture. The wire is usually easily removed under local anaesthesia. Bone plates should not be placed near the oral mucosa as they will tend to become exposed. Lower border wires sometimes give rise to pain and discomfort if the overlying skin is thin. In these circumstances they should be removed.

Bone plates, particularly the larger compression plates, may become infected some time after the fracture has healed. Surgical removal of the plate will lead to rapid resolution of the problem.

Sequestration of bone

Comminuted fractures of the mandible, particularly those caused by missile injuries, may be complicated by the formation of bone sequestra. A sequestrum may be a cause of delayed union but often the fracture consolidates satisfactorily and the sequestrum remains as an actual or potential source of infection. Sequestra may then be extruded spontaneously into the mouth with quite minimal symptoms but sometimes a localized abscess forms and surgical removal of the dead bone becomes necessary. It is important to be sure that a sequestrum has separated completely from the healthy adjacent bone before surgical removal is contemplated. Very often an infection can be treated with antibiotics and the dead bone allowed to extrude spontaneously without surgical intervention.

Limitation of opening

Prolonged immobilization of the mandible in intermaxillary fixation will result in weakening of the muscles of mastication. If there has been substantial haemorrhage within muscles a considerable amount of organizing haematoma and early scar tissue may be present when fixation is released. All these factors combine to cause limitation of opening and a restricted mandibular excursion. In the majority of cases full movement is restored in time but as with other fractures, physiotherapy may accelerate the recovery period. Simple jaw exercises and mechanical exercisers may be employed with advantage. Occasionally manipulation of the mandible under anaesthesia may assist the breakdown of scar tissue within muscles.

Fibrodysplasia ossificans involving the main muscles of mastication is a very rare complication of mandibular fractures. It is believed that a haematoma occurs in the muscle, which organizes and eventually becomes ossified. That view is supported by the finding of trabecular bone within the muscle mass at subsequent operation (Narang and Dixon, 1974). Treatment consists of excision of the ectopic bone but the condition will often recur. The complication is extremely rare considering the frequency of mandibular injury and systemic factors may play a part in the disorder.

Scars

Many mandibular fractures have associated soft-tissue injuries and providing these wounds are carefully cleaned and sutured minimal scarring occurs. At first all scars tend to be red and feel hard to the touch but during the first year they soften and fade. Massage of the scar by the patient and the application of lanoline are very helpful in this respect. Occasionally hypertrophic scarring or keloid occurs producing an ugly deformity. Unsightly scars also result from contamination of the original wound with dirt, especially tar products. In all these circumstances surgical revision maybe beneficial but should not be contemplated until at least 1 year has elapsed. Unsightly scars can largely be prevented by adequate wound toilet and careful suturing of the original laceration.

Chapter 12

Fractures with gross comminution of bone and loss of hard and soft tissue

Although this type of mandibular fracture can occur in civilian practice from certain industrial injuries or injuries caused by fast-moving projectiles, it is more commonly associated with missiles employed in war or civil disturbance. The main differences between missile injuries of the mandible and the type seen in civilian practice can be enumerated as follows:

1. The fracture is usually extensively comminuted.
2. It is always compound and contaminated by foreign matter and bacteria.
3. The viability of the bone fragments and the extent of injury to teeth cannot be accurately evaluated preoperatively from clinical and radiographic examination.

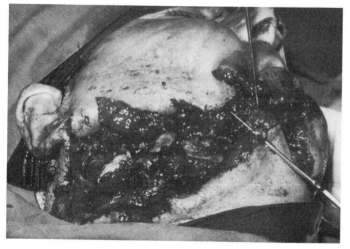

Figure 12.1 Intra-operative view of missile injury of the right mandible. The wound has been cleaned. Attached fragments of bone can be seen within the wound and the degree of skin loss can be appreciated. (Same case as illustrated in Figure 10.1 and reproduced by courtesy of Mr A. E. Brown)

4. Fracture treatment is complicated by soft-tissue injury or loss (Figure 12.1).

Bullets and other missiles travelling at high velocities cause this extensive damage because of the release of kinetic energy at the point of impact. Kinetic energy is proportional to the square of the velocity and it is therefore the impact velocity of the missile which is the most important factor. At impact there is deformation and sometimes fragmentation of the missile. The release of energy produces temporary cavitation within the tissues. These factors result in widespread damage adjacent to the missile tract and an 'explosive' exit wound although the entry wound may be comparatively small.

Such extensive injuries of the mandible require protracted treatment and the management can be divided into four main phases.

Immediate post-traumatic phase

The patient is not particularly shocked as a result of a facial injury alone but haemorrhage may be severe. These patients are often fully conscious even after extensive injury and maintain surprisingly good control over their own airway as they are able to position themselves so that blood and debris do not obstruct respiration. If consciousness is depressed immediate steps must be taken to remove blood and debris from the mouth and to control the tongue by a suture if necessary. Care must be taken in transporting such patients to ensure they are not laid on their backs in which position they may rapidly suffocate. Stretcher cases should be laid face downward with their face over the end of the stretcher and their forehead supported on a bandage tied between the two handles of the stretcher, or they can be carried lying on their side. Either position ensures that the tongue falls forward and blood and saliva drain out of the mouth. Ambulatory patients will spontaneously hold their face downward and forward.

These patients suffer surprisingly little pain and powerful analgesics which depress the cough reflex should not be administered.

Primary surgery

The surgical treatment of the fracture is often an incidental stage in the management of the wound as a whole. Often extensive wounds can only be managed after preliminary tracheostomy to ensure immediate and postoperative control of the airway. The stages of treatment will be as follows:

Wound toilet

A missile injury is always contaminated and intensive preliminary toilet is necessary in most cases, before formal surgical closure is undertaken.

Debridement

When the wound is ready for definitive surgery thorough debridement should be carried out to remove all devitalized tissue.

Management of involved teeth

Teeth are both a source of subsequent wound infection and a means of fixation. Their status in these two respects may only be determinable by inspection at the time of primary surgery. It is therefore very difficult to design fixation before the patient is under an anaesthetic. In general all extensively damaged and subluxed teeth should be removed. There are, however, occasions when temporary retention of damaged teeth may be necessary simply to control large loose alveolar fragments. Infection and delayed healing may result from such a decision in which case the involved teeth are removed at a later date by which time some consolidation of the bone fragments will have occurred.

Reduction and fixation

Every attempt must be made to establish bone continuity especially in the symphysis region. This can sometimes be achieved by deliberately displacing fragments to compensate for bone loss. Where irretrievable bone loss has taken place the remaining portions of the mandible should be positioned in their normal relationship and separately immobilized. In general arch wires provide the most versatile form of fixation assisted by a minimal number of transosseous wires.

Closure of mucosa and skin

The oral mucosa is closed first after the fracture has been suitably reduced and every attempt should be made to ensure that this closure is watertight. The jaws are then temporarily immobilized and the overlying skin wound is sutured. When skin loss has occurred it is often possible to obtain closure by undermining the wound edges or by raising local flaps. The rich vascular supply to the face permits the raising of local flaps from somewhat damaged tissue, whereas in other parts of the body similar flaps would undoubtedly fail. Skin to mucosa suturing should only be used as a last resort as it condemns the patient to extensive secondary reconstruction. Every effort must be made to reconstitute the oral sphincter even if this results in some distortion or reduction in size of the mouth orifice.

Drainage

Comminuted bone within a sleeve of healthy periosteum will heal in continuity. If, however, the periosteal sleeve becomes infected the fragments of bone will necrose and sequestrate leading to non-union. For this reason drains should be used liberally in contaminated comminuted fractures of the mandible. Through-and-through drains which allow subsequent irrigation of the fracture site are often helpful in preventing or controlling infection. It must be remembered that all wounds of the 'gunshot' type are infected from the outset however 'clean' they may appear after débridement.

Immediate postoperative phase

Patients who have sustained severe facial injuries of this nature are very conscious of their actual and potential deformity. They require sympathetic nursing to bolster their confidence. Special feeding devices may be needed if there is soft-tissue loss involving the oral sphincter and sometimes some form of saliva shield may have to be constructed to prevent the constant escape of oral secretions. Oral hygiene is, of course, even more important than in simpler fractures and the patients usually require active assistance with mouth irrigation. Tracheostomy management and care of wound drains need specialized nursing care to avoid serious complications.

Reconstructive phase

There is no doubt that surgical expertise in treating the original injury can do much to reduce the amount of later reconstruction.

If mandibular continuity is established even with considerable loss of mandibular thickness, function is restored more quickly and the need for later bone grafting avoided. Similarly, ingenuity in the use of local flaps during initial wound closure will minimize the effects of skin loss. Nevertheless some reconstruction is usually necessary. Skin may have to be brought in and bone contour modified or re-established. Teeth need to be replaced and many patients require special prostheses. The reconstructive phase of treatment of these extensive disfiguring injuries may involve numerous hospital visits and further operations over a considerable period of time.

Bibliography

Adams, W. M. and Adams, L. H. (1956) Internal wire fixation of fractures. 15-year follow-up. *Am. J. Surg.*, **92**, 12

Adekeye, E. O. (1980) The pattern of fractures of the facial skeleton in Kaduna, Nigeria: a survey of 1447 cases. *Oral Surg.*, **49**, 491

Adell, R., Eriksson, B., Nylen, O. and Ridell, A. (1987) Delayed healing of fractures of the mandibular body. *Int J. Oral Maxillofac. Surg.*, **16**, 15

Afzelius, L. and Rosen, C. (1980) Facial fractures: a review of 368 cases. *Int. J. Oral Surg.*, **9**, 25

Alty, H. M. (1963) Atrophy of the mandible and spontaneous fracture. *Br. Dent J.*, **114**, 188

Amaratunga, N. A. deS. (1988) A comparative study of the clinical aspects of edentulous and dentulous mandibular fractures. *J. Oral Maxillofac. Surg.* **46**, 3

Andreason, J. O. and Andreason, F. M. (1990) *Essentials of Traumatic Injuries to the Teeth.* Copenhagen, Munksgaard

Andrews, J. (1968) Maxillo-facial trauma in Vietnam. *J. Oral Surg.*, **26**, 457

Arentz, R. (1967) Severe facial fractures in a haemophiliac. *J. Oral Surg.* **25**, 358

Atterbury, R. A. and Panagopoulos A. P. (1959) Management of multiple, compound, comminuted mandibular fracture in a 3 year old child. *Oral Surg.*, **12**, 421

Awty, M. D. and Banks, P. (1971) Treatment of maxillofacial casualties in the Nigerian Civil War. *Oral Med. Oral Surg. Oral Pathol.*, **31** 4

Banks P. (1975) Fixation of facial fractures. *Br. Dent. J.*, **138**, 129

Banks, P. (1985) Gunshot wounds. In *Maxillofacial Injuries* (eds N. L. Rowe and J. Ll. Williams), Edinburgh, Churchill Livingstone

Battersby, T. G. (1966) Plating of mandibular fractures. *Br. J. Oral Surg.*, **4**, 194

Battersby, T. G. (1967) Sequel to gunshot wound of face. *Br. J. Oral Surg.*, **5**, 117

Battle, R. J. V. (1953) War history of plastic surgery in the army. *History of the Second World War (Surgery)*, p. 341. London, HMSO

Becker, H. L. (1979) Treatment of initially infected mandibular fractures with bone plates. *J. Oral Surg.*, **37**, 310

Becker, R. (1974) Stable compression plate fixation of mandibular fractures. *Br. J. Oral Surg.*, **12**, 13

Becker, W. H. (1950) Transosseous wiring fixation of condylar fractures with intrafacial incision. *Oral Surg.*, **3**, 284

Becker, W. H. (1952) Open reduction of mandibular fractures. *Oral Surg.*, **5**, 447

Beckler, A. E. and Walker, R. V. (1969) Condylar fractures. *J. Oral Surg.*, **27**, 563

Bisi, R. H. (1973) The management of mandibular fractures in edentulous patients by intramedullary pinning. *Laryngoscope, St Louis, **83**, 22

Blevins, C. and Gores, R. J. (1961) Fractures of the mandibular condyloid process: results of conservative treatment in 140 patients. *J. Oral Surg.*, **19**, 392

Block, C. *et al.* (1972) Use of a metal intra-osseous fixation device for treatment of fractures of atrophic edentulous mandibles. *J. Sth. Calif. Dent. Assoc.*, **40**, 996

Booth, N. A. (1953) Complications associated with treatment of traumatic injuries of the oral cavity: aspiration of teeth. *J. Sth. Calif. Dent. Assoc.*, **11**, 242

Bosco, H. F. (1960) Reconstruction of mandible following bone loss due to osteomyelitis in the line of fracture. *Oral Surg.*, **13**, 663

Bottcher, Von M., Schonberger, A. and Sumnig, W. (1988) Erfoldsbewertung konservativer und chirurgischer Therapiemethoden bei Keifergelenfrakturen. *Zahn- Mund- Keiferheilk. Vortr.*, **76**, 283

Boyne, P. J. (1967) Osseous repair and mandibular growth after subcondylar fractures. *J. Oral Surg.*, **25**, 300

Bradley, J. C. (1972) Age changes in the vascular supply of the mandible. *Br. Dent. J.*, **132**, 142

Bradley, J. C. (1975) A radiological investigation into the age changes of the inferior dental artery. *Br. J. Oral Surg.*, **13**, 82

Bradley, P. (1985) Injuries of the condylar and coronoid process. In *Maxillofacial Injuries* (eds N. L. Rowe and J. Ll. Williams), Edinburgh, Churchill Livingstone

Bradnum, P. (1960) Improved method of fixation of silver splints. *Br. Dent. J.*, **108**, 302

Bramley, P. and Forbes, A. (1960) A case of progressive hemiatrophy presenting with spontaneous fractures of the lower jaw. *Br. Med. J.*, **1**, 1476

Broadbent, T. R. (1954) Mandibular condyle fractures. *Plast. Reconstr. Surg.*, **14**, 148

Bromidge, M. R. (1971) Severe compound comminuted fractures of the mandible. *Br. J. Oral Surg.*, **9**, 29

Brons, R. (1970) *Stabiele Interne Fixatie bij Corpus Mandibulae-Frakturen.* Groningen, Niemeyer

Brook, I. M. and Wood, M. (1983) Aetiology and incidence of facial fractures in adults. *Int. J. Oral Surg.*, **12**, 293

Brown, A. E. and Obeid, G. (1984) A simplified method for the internal fixation of fractures of the mandibular condyle. *Br. J. Oral Surg.*, **22**, 145

Brown, J. (1981) Enteral feeds and delivery systems. *Br. J. Hosp. Med.*, **26**, 168

Brown, J. B., Fryer, M. P. and McDowell, F. (1949) Internal wire-pin immobilization of jaw fractures. *Plast. Reconstr. Surg.*, **4**, 30

Brown, J. B. and McDowell, F. (1942) Internal wire fixation for fractures of the jaw: preliminary report. *Surg. Gynecol. Obstet.* **74**, 227

Bruce, R. A. and Strachen, D. S. (1976) Fractures of the edentulous mandible: Chalmers J. Lyons Academy study. *J. Oral Surg.*, **34**, 973

Bruksch, K. Effect of intermaxillary fixation on ventilatory capacity. *MS Thesis*, University of Minnesota

Burch, R. J. *et al.* (1958) Method of reduction for impacted and partially malunited fractures of the jaws. *J. Oral Surg.*, **16**, 336

Busuito, M. J., Smith, D. J. and Robson, M. C. (1986) Mandibular fractures in an urban trauma centre. *J. Trauma*, **26**, 826

Buxton, J. L. D., Parfitt, G. J. and MacGregor, A. N. (1941) Arch wires for the immobilization of fractures of the mandible. *Br. Dent. J.*, **71**, 295

Byrne, R. P. (1972) Occult fracture of the odontoid process: report of case. *J. Oral Surg.*, **30**, 684

Calhoun, N. R. and Perkins, R. L. (1958) Compound, comminuted fracture of body of mandible. *J. Oral Surg.*, **16**, 510

Campbell, W. (1977) Radiological evaluation of facial fractures. Lesson 39, in *Weekly Radiology Science Update.* Narberth Pennsylvania, Biomedia Inc.

Cawood, J. I. (1985) Small plate osteosynthesis of mandibular fractures. *Br. J. Oral Maxillofac. Surg.*, **23**, 77

Champy, M. and Lodde, J. P. (1977) Etudes des contraintes dans la mandibule fracturée chez l'homme: mesures theoriques et verification par jauges extensometriques in situ. *Rev. Stomatol. Chir. Maxillofac. (Paris)*, **78**, 545

Champy, M., Lodde, J. P., Schmitt, R., Jaeger, J. H. and Muster, D. (1978) Mandibular osteosynthesis by miniature screwed plates via a buccal approach. *J. Maxillofac. Surg.*, **6**, 14

Charlton, H. (1967) An occipital air support for use with the Ellis 'Halo'. *Br. J. Oral Surg.*, **5**, 167

Ching, M. and Hase, M. P. (1987) Comparison of panoramic and standard radiographic radiation exposures in the diagnosis of mandibular fractures. *Med. J. Aust.*, **147**, 226

Choukas, N. C. *et al.* (1970) Effects of surgically reduced fracture dislocations of mandibular condyles on facial growth in Macaca Rhesus monkeys. *J. Oral Surg.*, **28**, 113

Chuong, R. and Piper, M. A. (1988) Open reduction of condylar fractures of the mandible in conjunction with repair of discal injury. *J. Oral Maxillofac. Surg.*, **46**, 257

Clarkson, P. W., Wilson, T. H. H. and Lawrie, R. S. (1946) Treatment of 1000 jaw fractures. *Br. Dent. J.*, **80**, 69

Cohen, B. (1968) Management of comminuted mandibular fractures. *J. Oral Surg.*, **26**, 537

Cohen, L. (1960) Further studies into the vascular architecture of the mandible. *J. Dent. Res.*, **39**, 936

Curran, J. B. *et al.* (1972) Diplopia as a sign of basal skull fracture accompanying a fractured mandible: report of case. *J. Oral Surg.*, **30**, 845

Dahlstrom, L., Kahnberg, K.-E. and Lindahl, L. (1989) 15 years follow-up on condylar fractures. *Int. J. Oral Maxillofac. Surg.*, **18**, 18

De'Champlain, R. W. (1973) Mandibular reconstruction. *J. Oral Surg.*, **31**, 448

Des Prez, J. D. and Kiehn, C. L. (1959) Methods of reconstruction following resection of anterior oral cavity and mandible for malignancy. *Plast. Reconstr. Surg.*, **24**, 238

Dingman, R. O. and Alling, C. C. (1954) Open reduction and internal wire fixation of maxillo-facial fractures. *J. Oral Surg.*, **12**, 140

Dingman, R. O. and Harding, R. L. (1951) Treatment of mal-union of fractures of the facial bones. *Plast. Reconstr. Surg.*, **7**, 505

Dingman, R. O. and Natvig, P. (1964) *Surgery of Facial Fractures.* Philadelphia, Saunders

Ditchfield, A. (1960) Interosseous wiring of mandibular fractures: a follow-up of 50 cases. *Br. J. Plast. Surg.*, **13**, 146

Donoff, R. B. *et al.* (1973) Management of condylar fractures in patients with cervical spine injury: report of cases. *J. Oral Surg.*, **31**, 130

Down, M. G. (1972) Indirect skeletal fixation. *Br. J. Oral Surg.*, **10**, 35

Ellis, D. *et al.* (1972) Fracture of the mandible in a 5-year-old infant. *Oral Surg.*, **33**, 348

Ellis, E., Moos, K. F. and El Attar, A. (1985) Ten years of mandibular fractures: an analysis of 2137 cases. *Oral Surg.*, **59**, 120

El-Mofty, S. (1972) Ankylosis of the temporomandibular joint. *Oral Surg.*, **33**, 650

Eriksson, L. and Willmar, K. (1987) Jaw fractures in Malmo 1952–62 and 1975–85. *Swed. Dent. J.*, **11**, 31

Farish, S. E. (1972) Iatrogenic fracture of the coronoid process: report of case. *J. Oral Surg.*, **30**, 848

Fickling, B. W. (1946) Advances in construction and use of splints in treatment. *Br. Dent. J.*, **80**, 8

Fordyce, G. L. (1957) Pyriform aperture wiring in the treatment of mandibular fractures. *Br. J. Plast. Surg.*, **9**, 304

Freihofer, H. P. M. (1973) Experiences with intra-oral transosseous wiring of mandibular fractures. *J. Maxillofac. Surg.*, **1**, 248

Fry, W. K. (1929) Fractures of the mandible in and posterior to the molar region. *Proc. R. Soc. Med.*, **22**, 37

Fry, W. K., Shepherd, P. P., McLeod, A. C. and Parfitt, G. J. (1943) *The Dental Treatment of Maxillo-facial Injuries*. Oxford, Blackwell

Fryer, M. P. (1971) Evaluation of internal wire pin fixation of mandibular fractures. *Surg. Gynecol. Obstet.*, **132**, 19

Fuhr, K. and Setz, D. (1963) Nachuntersuchengen uber Zahne die zum Bruchspalt in Beziehung stehen. *Dtsch. Zahnaertztl. Z.*, **18**, 638

Gariulo, E. A. (1973) Use of titanium mesh and autogenous bone marrow in the repair of a non-united mandibular fracture: report of case and review of the literature. *J. Oral Surg.*, **31**, 371

Georgiade, N. G. (ed.) (1969) *Plastic and Maxillo-facial Trauma Symposium*. St Louis, Mosby

Gerry, R. G. (1965) Condylar fractures. *Br. J. Oral Surg.*, **3**, 114

Gilhuus-Moe, O. (1971) Fractures of the mandibular condyle in the growth period. *Acta Odontol. Scand.*, **29**, 53

Gillies, H. D. (1920) *Plastic Surgery of the Face*. London, Oxford University Press

Glineberg, R. W., Laskin, D. M. and Blaustein, D. J. (1982) The effects of immobilisation on the primate temporomandibular joint. A histologic and histochemical study. *J. Oral Maxillofac. Surg.*, **40**, 3

Goin, D. W. (1980) Facial nerve paralysis secondary to mandibular fracture. *Laryngoscope*, **90**(11), 1777

Goodsell, O. (1964) Traumatic myositis ossificans of the masseter muscle. *Br. J. Oral Surg.*, **2**, 137

Goracy, E. S. *et al.* (1971) Traumatic refracture of the mandible. *Oral Surg.*, **32**, 378

Gordon, S. (1957) A prosthetic mandibular head: case report. *Plast. Reconstr. Surg.*, **20**, 62

Gorman, J. M. *et al.* (1972) An impacted mandibular fracture. *Br. J. Oral Surg.*, **10**, 95

Grattan, E. (1972) Patterns, causes and prevention of facial injury in car occupants. *Proc. R. Soc. Med.*, **65**, 913

Grattan, E. and Hobbs, J. A. (1985) Applied surgical anatomy: mechanisms of injury to the face in road traffic accidents. In *Maxillofacial Injuries* (eds N. L. Rowe and J. Ll. Williams), Edinburgh, Churchill Livingstone

Gunning, T. B. (1866) The treatment of fractures of the lower jaw by interdental splints. *N. Y. Med. J.*, **3**, 433

Halazonetis, J. A. (1968) The weak regions of the mandible. *Br. J. Oral Surg.*, **6**, 37

Hanratty, W. J. and Naeve, H. F. (1964) Actinomycosis with pathologic fracture of mandible. *Oral Surg.*, **18**, 303

Harnisch, H. (1959) Five-year statistics of jaw fractures. *Zahnärztl. Prax.*, **10**, 126

Hendrik, J. H., Sanders, S. G., Green, B. *et al.* (1959) Open reduction of mandibular condyle; a clinical and experimental study. *Plast. Reconstr. Surg.*, **23**, 283

Hirschfelder, U., Mussig, D., Zschiesche, S. and Hirschfelder, H. (1987) Funktionskieferorthopadisch behandelte Kondylusfrakturen – eine klinische und computertomographische Untersuchung. *Fortschr. Kieferorthop.*, **48**, 504

Hohl, T. H., Shapiro, P. A., Moffett, B. C. and Ross, A. (1981) Experimentally induced ankylosis and facial asymmetry in the Macaque monkey. *J. Maxillofac. Surg.*, **9**, 199

Holden, M. (1968) An unusual complication arising during the treatment of a mandibular fracture. *Br. J. Oral Surg.*, **6**, 93

Hoopes, J. E. *et al.* (1970) Operative treatment of fractures of the mandibular condyle in children using the post-auricular approach. *Plast. Reconstr. Surg.*, **46**, 357

Howe, G. L. and Wilson, J. S. P. (1964) Traumatic arterio-venous aneurysm occurring as a complication of a mandibular fracture: case report. *Br. J. Oral Surg.*, **2**, 54

Huelke, D. F. and Burdi, A. R. (1964) Location of mandibular fractures related to teeth and edentulous regions. *J. Oral Surg.*, **22**, 396

Huelke, D. F., Burdi, A. R. and Etyman, C. E. (1961) Mandibular fractures as related to the site of trauma and the state of dentition. *J. Dent. Res.*, **40**, 1262

Huelke, D. F. and Compton, C. P. (1983) Facial injuries in automobile crashes. *J. Oral Maxillofac. Surg.*, **41**, 241

Huelke, D. F. *et al.* (1962) Association between mandibular fractures and site of trauma, dentition and age. *J. Oral Surg.*, **20**, 478

Hueston, J. T. (1959) Surgical exposure of the dislocated mandibular condyle. *Br. J. Plast. Surg.*, **12**, 275

Hungerford, R. W. and Munsat, T. L. (1965) Mandibular fracture and myotonic dystrophy. *Oral Surg.*, **18**, 121

Hunsuck, E. (1967) A method of intraoral open reduction of fractured mandibles. *J. Oral Surg.*, **25**, 233

Hunter, K. M. (1972) Midline and condylar fracture in an 18-month-old child. *Aust. Dent. J.*, **17**, 373

Hut, M. (1960) Methods and appliances for the reduction and fixation of fractures of the facial bones. *Int. Dent. J., Lond.*, **10**, 468

Hutzschenreuter, P., Perren, S. M., Steinemann, S. *et al.* (1969) Some effects of rigidity of internal fixation on the healing pattern of osteotomies. *Injury*, **1**, 77

Irby, W., B. (1958) Correction of malreduced fractures of mandible at angles. *Oral Surg.*, **11**, 26

Irby, W. B. (1969) Facial injuries in military combat. Intermediate care. *J. Oral Surg.*, **27**, 548

Jacobsen, P. U. (1972) Unilateral overgrowth and remodelling processes after fracture of the mandibular condyle: a longitudinal radiographic study. *Scand. J. Dent. Res.*, **80**, 68

James, D. R. (1976) Atrophy of the mandible: reconstruction following fracture. *Br. J. Oral Surg.*, **14**, 156

James, R. B., Fredrickson, C. and Kent, J. N. (1981) Prospective study of mandibular fractures. *J. Oral Surg.*, **39**, 275

James, W. W. and Fickling, B. W. (1940) *Injuries of Face and Jaws*. London, Bale & Staples

Johansson, B., Krekmanov, L. and Thomsson, M. (1988) Miniplate osteosynthesis of infected mandibular fractures. *J. Craniomaxillofac. Surg.*, **16**, 22

Johnson, G. B. (1962) Multiple severe automotive injuries. Evaluation and management. *NC Med. J.*, **22**, 335

Jones, N. B. (1970) Dietary needs of the oral surgery patient with comparison of dietary supplements. *J. Oral Surg.*, **28**, 892

Jones, R. Watson (1952) *Fractures and Joint Injuries*, 4th ed., vol. 1. Edinburgh, Livingstone

Juniper, R. P. and Awty, M. D. (1973) The immobilization period for fractures of the mandibular body. *Oral Surg.*, **36**, 157

Kahnberg, K. E. (1979) Extraction of teeth involved in the line of mandibular fractures. I. Indications for extraction based on follow-up study of 185 mandibular fractures. *Swed. Dent. J.*, **3**, 27

Kahnberg, K. E. and Ridell, A. (1979) Prognosis of teeth involved in the line of fracture. *Int. J. Oral Surg.*, **8**, 163

Kai Tu, H. and Tenbulzen, D. (1985) Compression osteosynthesis of mandibular fractures – a retrospective study. *J. Oral Maxillofac. Surg.*, **43**, 585

Kazanjian, V. H. and Converse, J. M. (1949) *The Surgical Treatment of Facial Fractures*. Baltimore, Williams & Wilkins

Kazanjian, V. H. and Converse, J. M. (1959) *The Surgical Treatment of Facial Injuries*, 2nd ed. Baltimore, Williams & Wilkins

Keen, R. R. (1971) Mandibular fracture in a small child. *Ill. Dent. J.*, **40**, 87

Kendell, B. D., Fonseca, R. J. and Lee, M. (1982) Postoperative nutritional supplementation for the orthognathic surgery patient. *J. Oral Maxillofac. Surg.*, **40**, 205

Keniry, A. J. (1971) A survey of jaw fracture in children. *Br. J. Oral Surg.*, **8**, 213

Kersten, T. E. and McQuarrie, D. G. (1975) Surgical management of shotgun injuries of the face. *Surg. Gynecol. Obstet.* **140**, 517

Key, J. A. (1932) Positive pressure in arthrodesis for tuberculosis of the knee joint. *South Med. J.*, **25**, 909

Khosla, M. and Boren, W. (1971) Mandibular fractures in children and their management. *J. Oral Surg.*, **29**, 116

Kiehn, C. L. *et al.* (1961) Management of fractures of the mandibular condyle. *J. Trauma*, **1**, 279

Killey, H. C. (19068) Maxillo-facial injuries. *Hospital Med.*, **2**, 917

Killey, H. C. (1974) *Fractures of the Mandible*. 2nd ed. rev. rep. Bristol, Wright, p. 13

Kline, S. N. (1973) Lateral compression in the treatment of mandibular fractures. *J. Oral Surg.*, **31**, 182

Kromer, H. (1952) Reprinted from *Norske Tandlaegeforen. Tid.*

Kromer, H. (1953) Teeth in the line of fracture: a conception of the problem based on a review of 690 jaw fractures. *Br. Dent. J.*, **95**, 43

Kwapis, B. W., Dryer, M. H., Knox, J. E. *et al.* (1973) Surgical correction of a mal-united condylar fracture in a child. *J. Oral Surg.*, **31**, 465

Lal, D. *et al.* (1959) Management of fractures of lower jaw in children. *Oral Surg.*, **12**, 1413

Lamberg, M. A. (1978) Maxillofacial fractures – an epidemiological and clinical study on hospitalised patients. *Proc. Finn. Dent. Soc.*, **74**, 113

Lapidot, A. (1962) Clinical survey of fractures of the mandible with special reference to early and controlled mobilization and its effects on fracture union. *Oral Surg.*, **15**, 518

Laskin, D. M. (1978) The role of the meniscus in etiology of post-traumatic temporomandibular joint ankylosis. *Int. J. Oral Surg.*, **7**, 340

Laws, M. (1967) Two unusual complications of fractured condyles. *Br. J. Oral Surg.*, **5**, 51

Leake, D. (1971) Long-term follow-up of fractures of the mandibular condyle in children. *Plast. Reconstr. Surg.*, **47**, 127

Leonard, M. S. (1987) The use of lag screws in mandibular fractures. *Otolaryngol. Clin. North Am.*, **20**, 479

Le Quesne, L. P. (1957) *Fluid Balance in Surgical Practice*, 2nd ed. London, Lloyd-Luke

Levin, H. L. (1965) Multiple fractures of the mandible with pathological connotations. *Oral Surg.*, **19**, 179

Lewis, G. K. and Perutsea, S. C. (1959) The complex mandibular fracture. *Am. J. Surg.*, **97**, 283

Lighterman, I. *et al.* (1963) Mandibular fractures treated with plastic polymers. *Arch. Surg., Chicago*, **87**, 868

Lindahl, L. (1977a) Condylar fractures of the mandible, I. *Int. J. Oral Surg.*, **6**, 12

Lindahl, L. (1977b) Condylar fractures of the mandible, IV. *Int. J. Oral Surg.*, **6**, 195

Lindahl, L. and Hollender, L. (1977) Condylar fractures of the mandible, II. A radiographic study of remodelling processes in the temporomandibular joint. *Int. J. Oral Surg.*, **6**, 153

Lindqvist, C. R., Kontio, A. and Santavirta, S. (1986) Rigid internal fixation of mandibular fractures – an analysis of 45 patients treated according to the ASIF method. *Int. J. Oral Maxillofac. Surg.*, **15**, 657

Lindstrom, D. (1960) A comparative survey of jaw fractures during the years 1948–1958. *Suom. Hammaslääk. Seur. Toim.*, **56**, 16

Luhr, H.-G. (1968) Zur stabilen osteosynthese bei Unterkeiferfracturen. *Dtsch. Zahnarztl. Zeitschr.*, **73**, 754

Lund, K. (1972) Unusual fracture dislocation of the mandibular condyle in a 6-year-old child. *Int. J. Oral Surg.*, **1**, 53

Lundin, K., Ridell, N., Sandberg, A. *et al.* (1973) One thousand maxillo-facial and related fractures of the ENT clinic in Gothenburg: a 2-year prospective study. *Acta Otolaryngol.*, **75**, 359

McDowell, F., Barrett-Brown, J., Fryer, M. P. *et al.* (1954) *Surgery of Face, Mouth and Jaws.* St Louis, Mosby, pp. 52–55, 71–72

McDowell, R. and Brown, J. B. (1952) Internal fixation of jaw fractures. *Arch. Surg., Chicago*, **64**, 665

MacGregor, A. J. (1963) Adjustable locking plate for sectional metal cap splints. *Dent. Practit.*, **13**, 341

MacGregor, A. J. and Fordyce, G. (1957) The treatment of fracture of the neck of the mandibular condyle. *Br. Dent. J.*, **102**, 351

McGuirt, W. F. and Salisbury, P. L. (1987) Mandibular fractures. *Arch. Otolaryngol. Head Neck Surg.*, **113**, 257

MacLennan, W. D. (1952) Consideration of 180 cases of typical fracture of the mandibular condylar process. *Br. J. Plast. Surg.*, **5**, 122

MacLennan, W. D. (1956) Fractures of the mandible in children under the age of 6 years. *Br. J. Plast. Surg.*, **9**, 125

MacLennan, W. D. and Simpson, W. (1965) Treatment of fractured mandibular condylar process in children. *Br. J. Plast. Surg.*, **18**, 423

MacLeod, A. C. R. and Shepherd, P. R. (1941) Cap splints. *Br. Dent. J.*, **71**, 267

Mallett, S. P. (1950) Fractures of the jaw. A survey of 2124 cases. *J. Am. Dent. Assoc.*, **41**, 657

Marciani, R. D. and Hill, O. (1979) Treatment of the fractured edentulous mandible. *J. Oral Surg.*, **37**, 569

Markey, R. J. (1974) Condylar trauma and facial asymmetry: an experimental study. *Thesis*, University of Washington, pp. 1–32

Markey, R. J., Potter, B. E. and Moffett, B. C. (1980) Condylar trauma and facial asymmetry: an experimental study. *J. Maxillofac. Surg.*, **8**, 38

Marlette, R. H. (1963) Submucoperiosteal wire fixation of mandibular fractures. *J. Oral Surg.*, **21**, 409

Marsden, J. L. (1964) Fracture of the mandible due to radicular and residual odontogenic cysts. *Br. J. Oral Surg.*, **2**, 71

Masureik, C. and Eriksson, C. (1977) Preliminary clinical evaluation of the effect of small electrical currents on the healing of jaw fractures. *Clin. Orthop.*, **124**, 84

May, M. *et al.* (1972) Closed management of mandibular fractures. *Arch. Otolaryngol.*, **95**, 53

May, M., Cutchavaree, A., Chadaratna, P. *et al.* (1973) Mandibular fractures from civilian gunshot wounds: a study of 20 cases. *Laryngoscope, St Louis*, **83**, 969

Merkx, C. A. (1971) Treatment of pseudo arthrosis of the mandibular body by a sliding bone graft. *Arch. Chir. Neerl.*, **23**, 273

Michelet, F. X., Deymes, J. and Dessus, B. (1973) Osteosynthesis with miniaturised screwed plates in maxillo-facial surgery. *J. Maxillofac. Surg.*, **1**, 79

Miller, R. and McDonald, D. (1986) Remodelling of bilateral condylar fractures in a child. *J. Oral Maxillofac. Surg.*, **44**, 1008

Moilanan, A. (1980) Experiment with supine panoramic X-ray equipment in the diagnosis of mandibular fractures. *Rontgenblaetter*, **33**, 588

Mommaerts, M. Y. and Engelke, W. (1986) Erfahrungen mit der Osteosynthese-Platte nach Champy/Lodde bei Unterkeiferfrakturen. *Dtsch. Zahn-Mund-, Keifer-, Gesichts-Chirur.*, **10**, 94

Mooney, J. W. *et al.* (1972) Use of wire sutures for fracture fixation. *Oral Surg.*, **34**, 21

Morgan, E. J. R. (1960) Unusual complication of fracture of the neck of the mandibular condyle. *Br. Dent. J.*, **108**, 329

Morris, J. H. (1949) Biphase connector, external skeletal splint for reduction and fixation of mandibular fractures. *Oral Surg.*, **2**, 1382

Mowlem, R., Buxton, J. L. D., MacGregor, A. N. and Barron, J. N. (1941) External pin fixation of fractures of the mandible. *Lancet*, **2**, 291

Muller, W. (1969) Haufigkeit, sitz und ursachen der gesichtsschadelfrakturen. In *Traumatologie in Kiefer-und Gesichtsbereich* (ed. E. Reichenback), Leipzig, Barth, pp. 47–58

Muška, K. (1968) Suspended fixation of the mandible. *J. Oral Surg.*, **26**, 172

Nahum, A. M. (1975) The biomechanics of maxillofacial trauma. *Clin. Plast. Surg.*, **2**(1), 59

Narang, R. and Dixon, R. A. (1974) Myositis ossificans: medial pterygoid muscle: a case report. *Br. J. Oral Surg.*, **12**, 229

Nash, E. S. and Addy, M. (1980) The use of chlorhexidine gluconate mouthrinses in patients with inter-maxillary fixation. *Br. J. Oral Surg.*, **17**, 251

Neal, D. C., Wagner, W. F. and Alpert, B. (1978) Morbidity associated with teeth in the line of mandibular fractures. *J. Oral Surg.*, **36**, 859

Norman, J. E. (1982) Post-traumatic disorders of the jaw joint. *Ann. R. Coll. Surg.*, **64**, 29

Obwegeser, H. L. and Sailer, H. (1973) Another way of treating fractures of the atrophic edentulous mandible. *J. Maxillofac. Surtg.*, **1**, 213

Oikarinen, V. J. and Lindqvist, C. (1975) The frequency of facial bone fractures in patients with multiple injuries sustained in traffic accidents. *Proc. Finn. Dent. Soc.*, **71**, 53

Oikarinen, V. and Malmstrom, M. (1969) Jaw fractures (1284 cases). *Suom. Hammaslääk. Seur. Toim.*, **65**, 95

Olson,B. A., Fonseca, R. J., Zeitler, D. L. *et al.* (1982) Fractures of the mandible: a review of 580 cases. *J. Oral Maxillofac. Surg.*, **40**, 23

Panagopoulos, A. P. (1957) Management of fractures of the jaws in children. *J. Int. Coll. Surg.*, **28**, 806

Panagopoulos, A. P. and Mansueto, M. D. (1960) Treatment of fractures of the mandibular condyloid process in children. *Am. J. Surg.*, **100**, 835

Paul, J. K. (1968a) Continuous arch bar. *J. Oral Surg.*, **26**, 114

Paul, J. K. (1968b) Intraoral open reduction. *J. Oral Surg.*, **26**, 516

Perkins, C. S. and Layton, S. A. (1988) The aetiology of maxillofacial injuries and the seat belt law. *Br. J. Oral Surg.*, **26**, 353

Perren, S. M., Huggler, A., Russenberger, M. *et al.* (1969) The reaction of cortical bone to compression. *Acta Orthop. Scand.* (Suppl.), **125**, 19

Pogrel, M. A. (1986) Compression osteosynthesis in mandibular fractures. *Int. J. Oral Maxillofac. Surg.*, **15**, 521

Prein, J. and Kellman, R. M. (1987) Rigid internal fixation of mandibular fractures – basics of AO technique. *Otolaryngol. Clin. North Am.*, **20**, 441

Proffit, W. R., Vig, K. W., Turvey, T. A. *et al.* (1980) Early fracture of the mandibular condyles. *Am. J. Orthod.*, **78**, 1

Quinn, J. H. (1968) Open reduction and internal fixation of vertical maxillary fractures. *J. Oral Surg.*, **26**, 167

Ranta, R. and Ylipaavalniemi, P. (1973) The effect of jaw fractures in children on the development of the permanent teeth and the occlusion. *Proc. Finn. Dent. Soc.*, **69**, 99

Raveh, J., Vuillemin, T., Ladrach, K. *et al.* (1987) Plate osteosynthesis of 367 mandibular fractures. *J. Craniomaxillofac. Surg.*, **15**, 244

Reitzik, M. and Schoorl, W. (1983) Bone repair in the mandible – a histologic and biometric comparison between rigid and semi-rigid fixation. *J. Oral Maxillofac. Surg.*, **41**, 215

Rhinelander, F. W. (1974) Tibial blood supply in relation to bone healing. *Clin. Orthop.*, **105**, 34

Ridell, A. and Astrand, P. (1971) Conservative treatment of teeth involved by mandibular fractures. *Swed. Dent. J.*, **64**, 623

Roberts, A. *et al.* (1973) Prognosis of odontoid fractures. *Acta Orthop. Scand.*, **44**, 21

Roberts, W. R. (1964) Case for mandibular plating. *Br. J. Oral Surg.*, **1**, 200

Robertson, D. M. and Smith, D. C. (1978) Compressive strength of mandibular bone as a function of microstructure and strain rate. *J. Biochem.*, **11**, 455

Robertson, J. H. (1963) Treatment of fractures of maxilla and mandible by resin cap splints. *Br. Dent. J.*, **114**, 321

Robinson, M. (1959) Diagnosis of mandibular fractures by auscultation with percussion. *Oral Surg.*, **12**, 173

Robinson, M. (1960) New onlay–inlay metal splint for the immobilization of mandibular fractures. *Plast. Reconstr. Surg.*, **25**, 77

Robinson, M. and Yoon, C. (1963) 'L' splint for the fractured mandible: a new principle of plating. *J. Oral Surg.*, **21**, 395

Robinson, M. *et al.* (1963) Sleeve over interosseous wire to aid immobilization of jaw fractures. *Plast. Reconstr. Surg.*, **32**, 557

Robinson, M. E. (1971) Delayed surgical-occlusal treatment of malocclusion and pain from displaced subcondylar fractures: report of case. *J. Am. Dent. Assoc.*, **83**, 639

Roed-Petersen, R. and Andreason, J. O. (1970) Prognosis of permanent teeth involved in jaw fractures. *J. Dent. Res.*, **78**, 343

Rowe, N. L. (1954) The basic principles of the treatment of maxillo-facial injuries. *J. R. Nav. Med. Serv.*, **40**, 111

Rowe, N. L. (1960) Mandibular joint lesions in infants and adults. *Int. Dent. J., Lond.*, **10**, 484

Rowe, N. L. (1968) Fractures of the facial skeleton in children. *J. Oral Surg.*, **26**, 505

Rowe, N. L. (1969) Non-union of mandible and maxilla. *J. Oral Surg.*, **27**, 520

Rowe, N. L. and Killey, H. C. (1952) Fractures of the facial skeleton. *Dent. Practit.*, **3**, 34

Rowe, N. L. and Killey, H. C. (1968) *Fractures of the Facial Skeleton.* Edinburgh, Livingstone

Sabey, B. E., Grant, B. E. and Hobbs, C. A. (1977) Alleviation of injuries by use of seat belts. *TRRL Supplementary Report*, 289

Salem, J., Lilley, G. E., Cutcher, J. L. and Steiner, M. (1969) Analysis of 523 mandibular fractures. *Oral Surg.*, **26**, 390

Sazima, H. J., Graaft, M. L., Fulcher, C. L. *et al.* (1971) Transoral reduction of mandibular fractures. *J. Oral Surg.*, **29**, 247

Schenk, R. and Willenegger, H. (1967) Morphological findings in primary fracture healing. *Symp. Biol. Hung.*, **7**, 75

Schilli, W. (1977) Compression osteosynthesis. *J. Oral Surg.*, **35**, 802

Schuchardt, K. N., Schwenzer, B., Rottke, E. N. and Lentrodt, J. (1966) Ursachen, Häufigkeit und lokalisation der frakturen des gesichtsschädels. *Fortschr. Keifer. Gesichtschir.*, **11**, 1

Schultz, R. C. (1973) The management of common facial fractures. *Surg. Clin. N. Am.*, **53**, 3

Seshul, M. B. *et al.* (1978) The 'Andy Gump' fracture of the mandible: a cause of respiratory obstruction or distress. *J. Trauma*, **18**(8), 611

Shelton, D. (1967) Study in wound ballistics. *J. Oral Surg.*, **25**, 341

Shepherd, J. P., Shapland, M., Pearce, N. X. and Scully, C. (1990) Pattern, severity and aetiology of injuries in victims of assault. *J. R. Soc. Med.*, **83**, 75

Shuker, S. (1985) Inter-rami intraoral fixation of severely comminuted mandibular war injuries. *J. Maxillofac. Surg.*, **13**, 282

Silk, D. B. A. (1980) Enteral nutrition. *Hospital Update*, **6**, 761

Song, I. C. *et al.* (1965) Anterior fixation of mandibular fractures. *Plast. Reconstr. Surg.*, **35**, 317

Sotham, J. C. *et al.* (1971) Structural changes around screws used in the treatment of fractured human mandibles. *Br. J. Oral Surg.*, **8**, 211

Souyris, F. *et al.* (1980) Treatment of mandibular fractures by intraoral placement of bone plates. *J. Oral Surg.*, **38**, 33

Spiessl, B. (1972) Rigid internal fixation of fractures of the lower jaw. *Reconstr. Surg. Traumatol.*, **13**, 124

Stephenson, K. L. and Graham, W. C. (1952) The use of a Kirschner pin in fractures of the condyle. *Plast. Reconstr. Surg.*, **10**, 19

Tansanen, A. and Lamberg, M. A. (1976) Transosseous wiring in the treatment of condylar fractures of the mandible. *J. Maxillofac. Surg.*, **4**, 200

Tashiro, H. and Notomi, K. (1979) The use of Kirschner wires in the treatment of low condylar fracture of the mandible. *Plast. Reconstr. Surg.*, **22**, 36

Taylor, D. V. (1966) Traumatic aneurysm and facial palsy as complications of a mandibular fracture. *Br. J. Oral Surg.*, **4**, 202

Thoma, K. H. (1948) *Oral Surgery*, vol. 1. London, Kimpton

Thoma, K. H. (1951) Transosseous wiring fixation of sub-condylar fracture. *Oral Surg.*, **4**, 290

Thoma, K. H. (1959) Treatment of jaw fractures, past and present. *J. Oral Surg.*, **17**, 30

Thoma, K. H. (1960) Progressive atrophy of the mandible complicated by fractures: its reconstruction. *Oral Surg.*, **13**, 4

Thomas, J. (1990) Road traffic accidents before and after seat belt legislation – study in a District General Hospital. *J. R. Soc. Med.*, **83**, 79

Thomson, H. G., Farmer, A. W., Lindsay, W. M. *et al.* (1964) Condylar neck fractures of the mandible in children. *Plast. Reconstr. Surg.*, **34**, 452

Treggiden, R., Wood, G. and Basha, E. G. (1973) Traumatic internal carotid artery occlusion following fracture of mandible. *Br. J. Oral Surg.*, **11**, 25

Upton, L. G. (1971) Modified healing in experimental mandibular fractures. *J. Oral Surg.*, **29**, 416

Van Hoof, R. F., Merkx, C. A., Stekelenburg, E. C. *et al.* (1977) The different patterns of fractures of the facial skeleton in four European countries. *Int. J. Oral Surg.*, **6**, 3

Vero, D. (1968) Jaw injuries. The use of Kirschner wires to supplement fixation. *Br. J. Oral Surg.*, **6**, 18

Vincent-Townend, J. R. L. and Langdon, J. (1985) Apendix to *Maxillofacial Injuries* (eds N. L. Rowe and J. Ll. Williams), Edinburgh, Churchill Livingstone

Wagner, W. F., Neal, D. C. and Alpert, B. (1979) Morbidity associated with extraoral open reduction of mandibular fractures. *J. Oral Surg.*, **37**, 97

Wald, R. M., Abemayor, E., Zemplenyi, J. *et al.* (1988) The transoral treatment of mandibular fractures using non-compression miniplates: a prospective study. *Ann. Plast. Surg.,* **20**, 409

Walker, D. G. (1957) Mandibular condyle: fifty cases demonstrating arrest in development. *Dent. Pract.,* **7**, 160

Walker, G., Harrigan, W., Rowe, N. L. and Walker, R. (1969) Clinical pathological conference on facial trauma. *J. Oral Surg.,* **27**, 575

Walker, R. V. (1960) Traumatic mandibular, condylar fracture dislocations. Effect on growth in the Macaca Rhesus monkey. *Am. J. Surg.,* **100**, 850

Wessberg, G. A., Schendel, S. A., Epker, B. N. *et al.* (1979) Monophase extraskeletal fixation. *J. Oral Surg.,* **37**, 892

Wheat, P. M., Evascus, D. S. and Laskin, D. M. (1977) Effects of temporomandibular joint meniscectomy in adult and juvenile primates. *J. Dent. Res.,* **58** (Special Issue) B, 139, Abstract 350

White, A. A., Punjabi, M. M. and Southwick, W. O. (1977) The four biomechanical stages of fracture repair. *J. Bone Joint Surg.,* **59A**, 188

Wilde, N. J. (1958) Malreduction, malposition and malunion in facial and mandibular fractures. *J. Int. Coll. Surg.,* **30**, 192

Williams, D. W. (1968) A modification of the eyelet wire. *Br. J. Oral Surg.,* **6**, 90

Williams, J. Ll. (1985) Nylon circumferential straps. In *Maxillofacial Injuries* (eds N. L. Rowe and J. Ll. Williams), Edinburgh, Churchill Livingstone, p. 332

Wilson, D. J. (1990) Imaging. In *A Textbook and Colour Atlas of the Temporomandibular Joint* (eds J. de B. Norman and P. Bramley), London, Wolfe Medical Publications Ltd, pp. 94–98

Wood, G. D. (1980) Assessment of function following fracture of the mandible. *Br. Dent. J.,* **149**, 137

Wood, G. D. (1981) The fractured condyle. *Dental Update,* p. 219

Wood, W. R., Hiatt, W. R. and Brooks, R. L. (1979) A technique for simultaneous fracture repair and augmentation of the atrophic edentulous mandible. *J. Oral Surg.,* **37**, 131

Worthington, P. and Champy, M. (1987) Monocortical miniplate osteosynthesis. *Otolaryngol. Clin. North Am.,* **20**, 607

Yaillen, D. M., Shapiro, P. A., Luschei, E. S. and Feldman, G. R. (1979) TMJ meniscectomy: effects on joint structure and masticatory function in *Macaca fascicularis. J. Maxillofac. Surg.,* **7**, 255

Yrastorza, J. A. and Kruger, G. O. (1963) Polyurethane polymer in the healing of experimentally fractured mandibles. *Oral Surg.,* **16**, 978

Zambito, R. F. and Laskin, D. M. (1964) Follicular cyst of mandible associated with pathologic fracture. *J. Oral Surg.,* **22**, 449

Zecha, J. J. (1977) Mandibular condyle dislocation into the middle cranial fossa. *Int. J. Oral Surg.,* **6**, 141

Zide, M. F. and Kent, J. N. (1983) Indication for open reduction of mandibular condylar fractures. *J. Oral Maxillofac. Surg.,* **41**, 89

Index